THE AGE OF HEALING:
PROFILES FROM AN ENERGY HEALER

THE AGE OF HEALING:
PROFILES FROM AN ENERGY HEALER

Neal Bogosian

With Forwards by Richard Gordon,
Founder of Quantum-Touch
and Alain Herriott

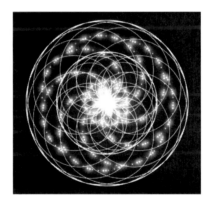

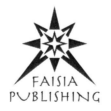

FAISIA
PUBLISHING

The information contained in this book is intended to be
educational and not for diagnosis, prescription, or treatment of any
health disorder or medical problem whatsoever. This information
should not replace consultation with a competent healthcare
professional and/or physician, either directly or indirectly. The
content of this book is intended for general information purposes
only, to be used as an adjunct to a rational and responsible health
care program prescribed by a health care practitioner. The author
and publisher are in no way liable for any misuse of the material.
Any application of the material set forth in the following pages is at
the reader's discretion and is his or her sole responsibility.

Author's website: www.quantumenergytreatment.com
Facebook: "The Age of Healing: Profiles from an Energy Healer"

ISBN-13: 978-0692439265
ISBN-10: 0692439269

Acknowledgements

I wish to thank the following people for their varying degrees of time, attention or inspiration: Richard Gordon, Author and Founder of *Quantum-Touch*; Jennifer Taylor, Chief "Magical" Officer (CEO) of *Quantum-Touch*; Alain Herriott, Author, Teacher and Healer; Tracy Cordner – for your initial editing expertise and feedback on the first draft of this book; Kimberly Carter Gamble, for your insights; Denise Rafkind of *Denise Rafkind Photography*, for your generous and amazing photo shoot and graphic design contributions; Goa Lobaugh, *Liquid Buddha Studios*; Kasia Wezowski; Andy McWain; my mother and father – Harry and Eileen Bogosian – for their constant love and support, and to Divine Spirit, Angelic friends, and guides... thank you for being my ever-present, ever-faithful teachers. *My life is my constant classroom. I hope I have pleased you.*

"A healthy body is the guest-chamber of the soul; a sick, its prison."

Francis Bacon, *Augmentis Scientiarum: Valetudo*

"Say you are well, or all is well with you, And God shall hear your words and make them true."

Ella Wheeler Wilcox, *Speech*

Contents

Energy Healing is the intended manipulation of Life Force energy and the influencing of the body energy systems, for the purpose of restoring the body to a state of well-being. It raises the energetic vibration and frequency of the body, so it can return to wellness, and heal itself; it is a natural meeting and amplification of energies between client and practitioner.

Forward

I've been in the field of energy healing for the past 40 years, and it's wonderful to see a wide range of "miraculous" sessions documented in a heartfelt and beautiful way. To the uninitiated, what Neal speaks of may seem to be impossible, a fantasy, or perhaps magic. Arthur C. Clarke wrote, "Any sufficiently advanced technology is indistinguishable from magic." But this is not magic, these are highly teachable skills that anyone can learn.

From my experience this kind of healing goes way beyond suggestion or any sort of placebo. We've seen this working on infants, animals, people under general anesthesia, plants, fluids, and even minerals. When I interview my advanced students, I hear a wide range of stories, which are exactly the sort that Neal tells. But since this sort of thing is so far outside of the comfort zone of most physicians and scientists, it is generally ignored or dismissed. The good news is that you don't need to believe in the ocean to get wet, you just need to jump in. When people take the leap and learn to use the energy of focused and amplified love, miracles abound.

Truly, with love and sincerity, nearly anything is possible. This is the take away from Neal Bogosian's inspiring book, "The Age of Healing: Profiles from an Energy Healer". Thank you.

Richard Gordon
Author/Founder of *Quantum-Touch*
Founder of *Self-Created Health*

Energy healing is about the application of consciousness both on the physical and spiritual level. We receive a session from someone and we are changed. Many will ask how this can be. Well, herein you will find many examples of how positive change can occur in seemingly impossible ways.

Neal has done a masterful job of presenting a series of cases to help everyone see that we are more than what appears on the surface. As he says, we are unlimited beings. When we are given an opportunity to have this divine spark lit, then amazing things occur. We change and this change fills us with hope and the willingness to dream a larger world that we can now explore. It is said, when the student is ready the teacher will appear. This book is a bridge and there are teachers everywhere to show you this or a similar path. If you are willing to step into the unknown, to explore the depths of new territory then you too can experience seeming miracles in your life. With time you will realize they are everyone's birthright.

> Alain R Herriott, author of *Supercharging Quantum-Touch*, *Quantum-Touch Core Transformations*, and the soon to be released, *The Art of Energy Healing and Awakening Through Wonder*

Introduction

We Are So Much More

I was inspired to write this book for a myriad of reasons large and small, which I will attempt to illuminate. One of the most significant reasons was the limited way that we, as a society, have been living our lives for a very long time; in our belief patterns, our disempowering dependence on people and institutions, and our lack of imagination and foresight. As we fully immerse ourselves in the 21st century, it can be said that Energy Healing is still an emergent, pioneering science, whose boundaries are still unknown. Many in our society have never heard of Energy Healing or Holistic Therapy. They remain unfamiliar with the entire modality, and vastly unaware of its amazing benefits. Others, who are deeply embedded in Western traditional medicine and its modern ways, are programmed to believe that pharmaceuticals, chemicals and surgery are the only ways to be fixed, healed and cured; they view Energy Healing as taboo. Some even suggest that anything "unknown" is from the devil, as if we were still living in the 16th century! This is to assume outright that we as humans do not have any powers within ourselves; that we must always rely on others for our wellness, or industries, machines, governments and institutions outside of ourselves. This cannot be further from the truth, and with regards to "truth", I have learned that what we perceive – or have perceived – to be "true", for the better part of the 19th and 20th centuries…is not true at all. New science and studies continue to emerge that contradict what were accepted as traditional truths, and with the expanse of the internet, every year brings "new" information in health and nutrition, purportedly outdating and poking holes in studies that were just done the year prior.

Thus, it is easy to confuse "content" with "truth". What is truth? Truth is often relative; it comes from within. Regarding healthcare, your truth – or what works for you and your body based on your experiences – may be different from mine and those around you, and that's okay. Mainstream humanity has unfortunately made it a habit to listen to others, accept their words, and believe that everything that is said and told is true; we have become very good servants, stripping ourselves of our own innate powers and talents. We have, for the most part, stifled our own ability to listen and to discern our *own* truth, surrendering this power to the words of others and what they tell us to believe as fact.

What is *true* ought to first emanate from within because our truth is always within us – it always has been, along with a treasure trove of untapped power. Through Energy Healing, personal empowerment, better health and inner growth can be attained, along with transforming sensations of love and solitude. It is a power or life source that can be spread throughout the world, revolutionizing 19th and 20th century health-care practices and theories, while having a positive effect on human relations…because the energy is often rooted in goodness and love.

If we, as a collective world populous, learn and become accustomed to opening up our minds, more awareness will come, and perhaps enlightenment. More understanding will be acquired about what the composition of reality really is, and what it is *not*! We must learn to stop looking outside of ourselves for the answers, because everything we need *is* within.

For a variety of human-related reasons, the modern human species has been very slow to evolve. This, in part, has been the result of failing to adequately apply discernment and critical thought, to everything we hear or are *told* to believe; to know the difference between enlightened insights, mass-influenced information, and deception. Energy Healing has been in existence since the beginning of time; it has been here since the beginning of *everything*, because *everything* is energy. The Shamans used it. Tibetan Monks still use it and have for centuries, and it can be argued, according to scripture, that Jesus Christ also used it when he healed the multitudes. Saint Valentine, after whom Valentine's Day is named, is said to have been a healer, and I urge you to read the story about him and the healing of the jailer's daughter. It is widely reported that she was cured of blindness, but she was also cured of epilepsy, and the latter part of the healing happened from a distance – also known as "distance healing". In the 1970's, Energy Healing was often referred to as *The Laying on of Hands*, used to bring comfort to hospital patients and others in need. Today, it is being used to heal some soldiers experiencing post-traumatic stress disorder (PTSD), on patients in Oncology Wards, as well as in many other places where improved well-being and health are in demand. It is my personal wish that more people on our globe will continue to awaken to other alternatives for their health.

You may be immediately asking, *"So where's the proof of Energy Healing?"* Or you may be questioning, *"What kinds of issues can be healed"?* As you will read in the coming pages, as an Energy Healer I have had clients who were told by traditional doctors that there was not a cure for their ailment, and as a 'last resort' they came to see me and experienced a relief of their symptoms, and a release from their ailment. This does *not* imply that the doctor was at fault, for they treated according to what they knew, but that knowledge is limited, and can most often be fit into a nice square box, or a computer laptop. How many of your doctors now walk into the room to see you, holding a laptop, especially since the litany of changes and new regulations emanating from the Affordable Care Act? We are all collectively much more colorful, pulsating with energy, vitality and the wonders of our imagination, with endless variables, to be placed on a chart or a computer program that lists diagnoses; and with the exception of some antibiotics, we are much more than a prescription of chemical pills to mask the symptoms, after which we are often sent on our way. Collectively, this somehow dehumanizes and minimizes us, combining us into a collective mass, and forcing us to conform to a system – one that is often addictive. Western medicine is far from perfect. In 2014, a Senate panel was told that medical error was the third leading cause of death in the United States. Senator Bernie Sanders of Vermont was the chairman of the panel. It should soon become evident to the masses that there is a place for Alternative Medicine and Alternative Healing methods, right beside traditional and Western medical procedures; Alternative or Holistic Therapy complements traditional Western medicine, in virtually every facet. However, Alternative and Holistic Therapies are *not* intended to *replace* Western medicine.

Once you open yourself up to the untapped potential and powers within you, and realize that there is a never-ending trove of human potential always available to us, the discovery will be startling! You will begin to understand that there really are energy currents all around us and running through us, and that we have the power to direct them. It may also solidify your belief in alternative healing and/or energy healing. You will likely encounter fewer health issues or incidents, and thus less need for traditional and Western medicine. You will find yourself no longer fixated on pharmaceutical commercials and the litany of diseases "they" make sure we know of, and what to do "if" we contract them. Isn't it time that we stopped focusing on everything that is bad or dangerous and full of disease?

We are constantly flooded with possibilities of doom, danger and death. There is indeed money to be made by keeping people sick and/or immersed in a negative vibrational frequency. Therefore, you have a choice: You can *choose* to stop listening to, and stop accepting negativity into your life. Positive, wholesome and healthy vibrations and thoughts from within have immeasurable power, and should always be chosen over anything negative. These positive, wholesome and healthy vibrations and thoughts can also be the first steps in understanding the energy and power within us. I urge you all to open up, awake, and explore this power (if you are not already), for it can trump and transform anything negative…and make those 'bumpy' days much *less* bumpy, resulting in a happier *you* with healthier thought patterns! *Happiness really is a choice*! One major fallacy that must be addressed in the early goings of this book is the belief in "limits". The fact is there are no limits. We are limitless, and I will remind you of this again.

Relevant to the acceptance of Energy Healing in the West, I have, in my possession, a copy of *Fate Magazine*, dated *January, 1958*. On the back cover is an advertisement for none other than, *Yoga*! It mentions its benefits and overall worthiness as a healthy regimen. Yes, this is how long it has taken for Yoga to assimilate into

Western culture. At the time of its publication, the magazine was considered to be in the genre of the occult! Today, Yoga centers and classes abound across the western states and territories, giving innumerable benefits to all who participate. Would you classify Yoga as being of the "occult"? Let us hope it does not take 40 or 50 years for Energy Medicine and Holistic/Alternative Healing to assimilate fully into our culture. I suspect it will not, for there are new energies presently flooding the planet, designed to accelerate our collective awakening and conscious ascension. However, these do *not* come without a series of shifts.

At present, it cannot be argued that our earth and our lives are changing rapidly and in drastic measure. Earthquakes, tornadoes and hurricanes are on the rise, as are wildfires and volcanoes. The earth is moving, and while these aforementioned phenomena can be severely destructive, they are also "energy shifters", shifting frequency patterns the world over. What does this mean? Humankind is slowly, gradually and in subtlety, experiencing these same shifts. Few understand that we as humans would not be able to exist here on earth if the energy frequency that runs through us was not compatible with that which runs through the earth. In terms of energy healing...all of these shifting patterns are boons to the practice. Over the past year

alone, I have seen the power of my energy healing mul-
tiply exponentially.

Can energy healing *only* be used to heal and help humans? No. Experiments in "global coherence" prove
that energy healing can be effective on a global scale,
affecting the entire earth. Energy healing can be used
to affect weather patterns, improve the environment,
heal pets and nature, and yield more bountiful crops.

The energy signature or aural pattern around some
plants can rival those circumventing some animals.
This is not to diminish life in any way, but consider for
a moment what this could mean for diets, health, and
healing, and better understanding the properties of vital life force energy that compose plants and trees.
However, more importantly…it means that plants are
just as much alive, teeming with energy as we are, and
when we send and emit an energy frequency of love or
abundance, the plants and trees receive it – and respond – just as humans and animals do. Energy healing, when exercised from a wholesome and intently
pure place, is set in love, the highest emotional frequency; it can mend or accelerate the healing of any issue (conversely the healer can suffer immeasurably if
negative or sinister intentions or ulterior motives are
employed). It is said that eons ago, in a prior civilization called, Lemuria, no trees were ever destroyed or

cut down; they were in fact, revered and loved for the beauty and vital energy they emitted, and thus they were very much *alive*. It was a time when the air was pure and breezes temperate, when everything that we deem mystical and wondrous today...actually existed in full form. It is a place to which we might aspire to return. Lemuria was not a hypothetical place. It was real, purportedly existing where Easter Island is now.

Quantum Physics (simply defined as the *energy* states of atoms which can implicate multiple dimensions) is also *real*. It is the science of *now,* and it is time that it is taught in secondary schools across the country. We now know enough about it, thanks in large part to Max Planck, and since its principles alone elicit the imagination, it should be the new beacon for the minds of our young, sparking and introducing endless possibilities into their periphery and better equipping them for the 21st century. It should replace the uniform, stilted, stale and antiquated science we teach our young today, or rather, material we still call "science" that does nothing to activate the imagination – facts and figures that are all dull, and in some instances, no longer applicable in this new, evolving age of humanity. Sadly however, not many people can even tell you what Quantum Physics is, and the basic premise of what it entails – because it was never taught to them. I am also a certified public educator, and when I listed Quantum Physics as a focus for my state's required life-long learning program, one of the coordinators from the Board of Education exclaimed, *"What? What's this? Oh, my God! They're going to love this when they see it!"* I frankly did not know how to react. I queried to myself, *Am I not in academia?* There is a lack of foresight in curriculums today – or perhaps it is me just looking too far ahead, but I am not alone. Famed writer Ray Bradbury said, "The ability to fantasize is the ability to grow." Quantum Physics can be born in our minds; in our lush imaginations that are always ripe to be called into action, dripping with the wanton desire to expand, progress and create, because this is who we are. We are not one-dimensional creatures, but rather multi-dimensional. Let us again teach ourselves and our children the importance of fantasizing; of fascination, its inherent marvels, and urge one and all to imagine, for it is here where everything is born and anything is attainable, including harmonious health. In Quantum Physics, which is much of what is employed in energy healing, everything is possible – *EVERYTHING*!

The following profiles of my work as an energy healer are presented herein, to not only educate and further demonstrate the validity of this healing science, but also to broaden the horizons and collective minds of all of those who read it; all of those collective minds who may still be locked into believing that only the standard or traditional way of administering medical care is all there is and all there should be. To think in this manner is to place limits and boundaries around humankind. Again, we as humans are limitless, bound-less beings of light and love, capable of so much more than what we have been programmed, nudged and told to believe. *This is fact*. Remember, "We are made in *His* likeness," and so, if *He* is unlimited and boundless, we are also! It is time to awaken to our true capacities. It is my hope that my profiles of actual healing sessions and associated events that I have personally experi-enced, will enlighten you and bring a smile to your face, a revelatory smile that elicits a sense of relief, knowing that there really *is* more...and we really are much more powerful and amazing than what we may have been led *or told* to believe.

This is *not* a 'how to' book, but rather a book of client profiles and healing stories that demonstrate the effec-tiveness, validity and amazing beauty of holistic en-ergy healing. This book is also *not* the final answer to health, but rather part of the beginning of an expanded awareness to other forms of healing, and the unlimited potential of humanity. I have added explanation and afterthoughts within each profile, where I felt applicable, for the purpose of further insight or clarification. Some of the profiles that follow border on the supernatural, but *all* of them are spiritual, for we are energetic spiritual beings...always. We are beautiful and loved in dimensions far beyond this small, tiny, illusory physical plane! *You* are loved! What follows is for you, from my heart to yours.

-- Neal Bogosian, Rhode Island, March 2015

A note about the profiles: Out of respect for privacy and to maintain anonymity, I have altered certain characteristics of the subjects, along with other identifiable information that might be otherwise revealing. I will also alternate in reference to the individuals in each case, as either "the subject", "the client", or a chosen pseudonym.

** The information contained in this book is for informational purposes only, and should not be used to replace professional medical advice. Readers are responsible for how they choose to utilize this content, and also for any application of the material set forth in the following pages.*

This information should not be considered complete, nor should it be relied on in diagnosing or treating a medical condition. Content in this book does not contain information on all diseases, ailments, physical conditions or their treatment.

It is best to seek advice and attention from your physician or qualified healthcare professional. Always consult your physician before beginning a new treatment, diet or health and fitness program.

About Me

I am certified in *Quantum-Touch*™ levels I and II (www.QuantumTouch.com), which has provided me with an invaluable foundation, for which I am ever-grateful, and I am further grateful to its founder, Richard Gordon, for making the modality available to the public. I went on to further my understanding of energy and quantum, through extensive personal research and countless hours of live trials and application. I have maintained my own private Holistic Energy Healing practice since 2010 (www.QuantumEnergyTreatment.com). I was also on the staff of the *Integrated Care Program*, at *Women & Infants Hospital*, for the oncology ward.

I hold a double Master's Degree in Education (Elementary and Special Education); a Bachelor's Degree in Communications, and a degree from *The American*

Academy of Dramatic Arts. I am also the author of the novel, *The Adventures of Chip Doolin*. I pursued holistic energy therapy because I care about others...about you, and because *I believe* there is so much more; I believe the measurements of human capacity are incomplete. I have experienced the profound healing we are each capable of manifesting. My aim is to help remove the veil that has shrouded human potential.

PROFILE 1

"There is nothing we can do.
You are slowly going to go blind."

Can you imagine being told you might never see again? That one day you might be without the gift of vision and all its beauty? Tim, the client in this profile, was told by his doctor that he was slowly going blind. Imagine, if you can, being unable to see color, except through your memories. Imagine never being able to see the faces of your loved ones, autumn leaves falling off trees, or never again being able to watch another movie or television show. As doctors in traditional western medicine often do, they give absolute, conclusive statements based only on what they know; based only on the charts, models and history available to them. What about what they do *not* know? What about the powers associated with hope and belief?

When this client first came to me, he was desperate for answers. The most wonderful aspect that he possessed was that he refused to believe what the doctor had told him. He was already a believer in alternative medicine and alternative ways to heal the body. The official diagnosis was *retinitis pigmentosa*, a genetic and degenerative eye disorder in which there is damage to the retina. It is a disease that historically results in severe vision impairment and blindness. To add to the challenge, he held a job that required the focused use of his eyes on a daily basis.

Immediately following his very first energy healing treatment, which lasted for more than one hour, there was marked improvement in his vision. I had focused exclusively on sending energy through my hands, and into his eyes. He reported seeing sharper contrasts in colors and being able to see small objects on the floor – something he could not do before the session began.

In my initial consultation with him, he reported that he could not see the small figures or toys on the floor of his home, with which his children enjoyed playing. He also reported that he was unable to spot a small spider on the floor, of which his spouse had asked him to dispose. However, immediately following my first session with him, all of that changed…and began to reverse. Tim quickly scheduled subsequent visits with me. It was during these subsequent visits when we both realized that his eyes were not the only part of him that was to experience the effects of directed energy, intention, and healing.

With just about every one of my clients, when I administer a healing session, I incorporate a multitude of processes that directly access quantum realms or quantum physics, hence quantum energy. This is activated through my mind, which is like having an always ready-to-use quantum machine. The mind is an entity that is far, far more powerful than what we have been led to believe, and combined with the power of the heart, it can form an unstoppable force capable of *anything*.

Another aspect not to be overlooked, and one that surely aided in the results of this healing, was the subject's overwhelming power of *belief*. There is so much power in believing. If you would, think of a sport you may have played, in which you achieved a level of success, or something that you know you are good at, perhaps even considered an expert. Could you achieve success if you did not believe in yourself, and in your skills or aptitude in the field? Take for instance a professional football running back. When the ball is handed to him, do you think his natural thoughts are, *Forget it! I can't break through that line, that's impossible*?

No, of course not or he would not be in professional sports. Before he is even handed the ball, he instinctively *knows* and *believes* that he is good enough to break through any defensive line. Yet, many in our society still use the word "cannot" or "impossible" or more specifically, "I've never seen that done or cured so forget it, it will never happen". These words and phrases are self-defeating. They serve no one! However, shift the focus to empowerment and a world of positive possibilities emerge; the possibility of *anything*! I remember major league pitcher, Jeff Suppan, before starting a World Series game, telling a reporter how he visualized – in his mind – his desirable or intended performance *before* he went to the mound. While Jeff had what many would consider an *average* career in pro baseball, no one expected him to last 17 seasons and win 140 total big league games – not to mention start a World Series game! Pro golfer Jack Nicklaus would also visualize before every shot. When I was growing up, I believed in the possibility of anything. I instinctively knew that there was so much more that we were capable of doing; I knew there were so many unlocked secrets, and I wanted to unlock them all!

Tim, despite being given the label of "retinitis pigmentosa", refused to believe he was going to go blind.

He believed anything was possible, and his power of belief brought him to me, because what one seeks, if it is sought long enough with desire and earnest, will be attained, and like-minded people are also brought into the path. That too, is the power of our minds, and connected to the Law of Attraction. Tim was seeking a cure, and also someone who would believe in the possibility of anything with him. Our energies were kindred.

During his second visit two weeks later, with his eyes closed (as many clients' eyes often are) he reported seeing a myriad of beautiful, rotating colors, a relatively common effect in the world of energy healing, but one that signifies the absolute presence and circulation of energy; for the client, it is a magical and remarkable experience. Having fallen asleep for about half of the session, he also reported feeling completely relaxed, which was in contrast to his state before the treatment. Once again, following the treatment his vision was sharp and even more improved. He said that the effects of the first treatment lasted about one and a half weeks, at which time they began to fade. I suggested that we gauge the duration of the positive effects again, and schedule accordingly.

While I continued to work with him, I alternated between placing my hands on his head and also over his eyes, visualizing his eyes as being healed. Visualization is an extremely potent tool from which I derive countless benefits and results, and it is something I employ for all of my clients. It is for this reason that I believe a strong imagination on behalf of the healer, one without boundaries, is a major component to a successful healing. The broader, more prolific and detailed the imagination, its equivalence in the vastness and depth of the healing will often be achieved. Many artists might relate to this concept because it is the same place where inspiration is found. Thomas Edison, Henry David Thoreau, and Robert Louis Stevenson, amongst many others, have all referred to this in their own varying ways.

It was during my 3rd session with Tim, when he had an enlightening experience that left an indelible impression. Once again, the positive effects of the 2nd treatment lasted for about a week and a half. I then advised him that we should try three consecutive sessions on three consecutive days, to test whether filling the eyes with a maximum amount of energy would result in a longer duration of the positive effects. He agreed. I was intent on guiding him to wellness, igniting his body's capacity to heal itself, and I was intrigued with the possibilities. However, what occurred was something neither of us expected, although, since this work encompassed the depths of spirituality, I knew it was possible.

While running energy into him (I can feel this is happening on a physical level, when my hands begin to buzz and tingle), he began to twitch and jerk in certain areas of his body. These were not convulsing jerks. They were what I have come to know as blockages being lifted or released.

The energy being injected goes to the places it needs to, filling any voids. Since it is "source energy" it is "smart energy", and it simultaneously interacts with my overall intention that is to manifest a physical body that is whole, perfect and in harmony. Our bodies are intelligent systems and coupled with my energetic intent, both body and energy synergistically *know* what needs to occur for the restoration of wholeness and/or perfection. Since everything is energy, any ailment or illness is the result of an energy shortfall or blockage, stemming perhaps from stress, cellular memories, a physical accident or genetics/DNA.

While Tim's body experienced these energetic releases, I noted that his eyes were in REM state – he was asleep...or so I thought. After about twenty minutes, his body suddenly jerked again, and his upper torso completely lifted off the table and came back down. Following the session, I asked what he felt and experienced, as I do with all of my clients. He slowly shook his head in mild amazement.

"I saw you," he said. "I was up there watching you." He was pointing at the ceiling of the room.

"Really!"

"Yes! There was light all around you and I could see you working on me."

"You had an *out of body experience*. Did you feel your body jerk off the table?" I asked.

"I think so. I felt myself falling – "

"When you came back into your physical body..."

"Yes. Wow! It was really amazing," he said.

"How are your eyes?"

"Great!"

Following his next session, Tim informed me that he could see beams of light all around his eyes. They were very intense beams and he could feel the energy coming into his eyes, right through the centers. He said that his eyes were fine all day long and he could see everything.

During his next visit, the last of the group of three, the energy was so strong going into his eyes during the session that they began producing tears and streaming down the sides of his temples.

"The energy was so strong!" he said following the session. "It was almost too strong to even keep my eyes closed. It wasn't painful, it was just intense! I felt my eyes tearing."

I did not have to see him again for almost four weeks! He scheduled another three sessions to "amp up" the energy again, in his eyes. Prior to the next session he told me that he usually had difficulty driving at night, and even more so in stormy weather. During a recent rain storm at night, he was able to drive more than an hour without a single issue or difficulty. This was progress.

I also began employing mantras with him. I told Tim to say to himself over and over, "These eyes are perfect. My eyes are whole, perfect, strong and powerful," an affirmation often used by the late Charles Haanel, creator of *The Master Key System*. Mr. Haanel himself said that the spiritual eye is perfect! Speaking in terms of quantum, our spiritual, ethereal body – often referred to as our "body double" – is always perfect. Properties of this spiritual body can be accessed. It is another tool I employ during the healing sessions.

Tim could feel the effects of the affirmations, a mild form of self-hypnosis designed to tell the all-obeying and all-powerful subconscious mind that an ailment or malady is gone. The subconscious mind then sends these messages to the body...and the body listens and manifests accordingly. For Tim, the affirmations collectively strengthened and reinforced his ability to believe.

I advised him to offer gratitude for his eyes and the service they provide for him, and to send this gratitude directly from his heart. Our cells have a communication center. They *feel* gratitude and emotions just like we do. Think about it...if we are comprised of cells and we feel emotion, should not each individual cell register emotion as well, hence the term "cellular memory"?

Following this string of three consecutive sessions, I did not see the subject again for three months. Let us be reminded of what his doctor had told him. *"There is nothing we can do. You are slowly going to go blind."* While I cannot say nor profess that the subject's disease was cured, what I am comfortable admitting is that we managed to cease the deterioration and prove that there *was* something more that we could do, and he felt so much better as a result of it.

I continue to see the client periodically. However, the next time I saw him – about three months later – was not for his eyes at all, but rather for an ailing joint related to a sports incident, which literally cleared at the conclusion of the session. When I inquired about his eyes, he told me, "You know, I tell myself my eyes are fine, like you told me. I'm not focusing on them as much and they really have been fine. Our minds are powerful." Yes, they are. More and more evidence points to the realization that the world and our respective realities are determined by "mind". We live in a 'thought-driven' universe.

*   *   *

In a 2005 *Nature* journal article, Richard Conn Henry, Professor in the *Henry A. Rowland Department of Physics and Astronomy*, at The Johns Hopkins University, presented evidence for, and expounded upon the "The Mental Universe" in which we live:

According to Sir James Jeans: "the stream of knowledge is heading towards a non-mechanical reality; the Universe begins to look more like a great thought than like a great machine. Mind no longer appears to be an accidental intruder into the realm of matter...we ought rather hail it as the creator and governor of the realm of matter."...In his play *Copenhagen*, which brings quantum mechanics to a wider audience, Michael Frayn gives these word (sic) to Niels Bohr: "we discover that...the Universe exists...only through the understanding lodged inside the human head..."...Physicists shy from the truth because the truth is so alien to everyday physics…The Universe is entirely mental…One benefit of switching humanity to a correct perception of the world is the resulting joy of discovering the mental nature of the Universe. We have no idea what this mental nature implies, but — the great thing is — it is true.[1]

This excerpt dwarfs the stale and mainstream scientific model that society and culture has unfortunately adopted. It immediately antiquates our perceptions of science as primitive metal rockets being blasted into space. A mental/mind universe is also much more exciting. Consider the wealth of power that we really do have, and all this time most of us never knew. Think of the possibilities – they are endless, because *we* are unlimited. We are all creators, made in *His* Likeness. A quantum scientific revolution is at our doorstep that will come to define the 21st century. We have just entered the age of healing, an age that will slowly gain momentum, and only become more powerful.

PROFILE 2

"The kidney stone was gone. We couldn't find it!"

The subject in this profile came to me for relief from pain stemming from a kidney stone that he was scheduled to have removed by his doctor, just two days later.

"I'm getting pain all down my left side. I just want it to lessen until the surgery on Thursday," he said.

As soon as he settled onto my table for the session, I began raising the vibration and frequency of my own energy and directing it into him, through concentrated breathing and focus, sending it through my hands and into his body. However, my overall intention was not only to get *rid* of the pain, but rather to get *rid* of the kidney stone altogether. I set my visualization to seeing the stone literally disintegrate. I imagined blasting it with white and gold light energy, and renewing/reversing cellular patterns in the area. In my mind's eye, I could see fragments of the stone flying up and out in the form of butterflies – a pleasant, positive and thus powerful image. His pain quickly began to subside.

Some who read this account may be skeptically wondering whether "intention" and "imagination" can really be powerful healing tools that affect what we know as "physical matter". Indeed, they *are* powerful. Again, I defer to the untapped powers of our minds, and now is a good place to also begin mentioning "intention" in conjunction with the heart, since pure intention – a pure and sincere desire to help and to heal – is of the heart. There is nothing greater than "heart power". It is pure love.

Intention and imagination are elements of quantum physics, whereby the mind is expanded dimensionally, originating in that place where ideas, dreams and visions are born; a place Carl Jung called, "the substrata of our subconscious minds". What one thinks about, he/she brings about; molecules and atoms are literally activated and conjoined in unseen space, to bring about the "intended" result. One of the most basic examples of this that I can give, is something that almost everyone has experienced. Let's suggest you haven't heard from a friend or relative in at least a few months. You start "thinking" (intention) about this friend or relative, which elicits a mental "image" (imagination) associated with that thought, which is connected directly to cellular memories of that person. Sometime over the next 48 to 72 hours, this person calls you on the telephone. What is the first thing you say to them? "I was just thinking about you!" This is a layman's example of the power of our thoughts and images, the latter directly correlating with our ability to imagine. It is also a small example of quantum, as your thoughts are literally traveling through the space of this realm at mach speed, and reaching that person and connecting to *their* thoughts – directly summoning them in unseen space!

According to physicist Niels Bohr, "Everything we call real is made of things that cannot be regarded as real," this is because everything is energy, and it cannot always be seen, or even measured. However, just because you cannot see it…don't dismiss it. Even the Bible corroborates with the limitless value of what is unseen, in 2 Corinthians 4:18, "So we fix our eyes not on what is seen, but on what is unseen, since what is seen is temporary, but what is unseen is eternal."[2] The messages and truths of life are in our midst…but society has been too blinded by deception, ego and ignorance, to see them, believe them, and adopt them.

As I continued to work on my client with the label of "kidney stone", I also began to employ a simple, positive mantra on my own. I said to myself over and over: *It is gone! It is gone! The label of "kidney stone" is gone!* I continued to visualize the stone being blown to bits by the energy beams I was injecting. The subject commented that he felt intense heat in the area, where my hands were, as the pain continued to diminish.

Following the session, he got up off the table without effort. I asked how he felt and if there were any other experiences that he wished to share.

"I really don't feel the pain like I did," he said, touching his side. "It feels more like just an ache. I felt some movement down there too."

"What do you mean? What kind of movement?" I asked.

"Just...movement, like something moved. I also saw some colors flash in my eyes."

I advised him to drink plenty of water for the remainder of the day, and that the energy would continue to circulate for the next 48 to 72 hours. Water can act as a conductor for the energy that has been worked through the body.

Two days later, I received a phone call from his spouse.

"Neal?"

"Yes?"

"You're not going to believe it."

"What?"

"I am in the waiting room of the hospital. The doctor just came in. He had this dumbfounded look on his face. He looked at me and said, 'I can't really explain this. Uh...the kidney stone was gone. We couldn't find it. I saw where it *was* – where it was lodged against his kidney because there was some irritation at that spot, but the stone wasn't there, and he could not have passed it because it was too big to pass. I can't explain it. All I found was ash.' Do you believe it?" she finally asked.

"That's wonderful! And yes, I *do* believe it because I know what energy healing can do!"

"I told the doctor," she said.

"You told him what?"

"I told him we went to see you to get a Quantum Energy Treatment, and he said, 'Wow! Who is this guy? He may really be onto something here – I mean, he may *really* be onto something. I don't know where that stone went!'"

I burst into a happy laughter. "That's wonderful news! Thank you so much for calling to tell me."

"Well," she said, "whatever it is you do...it works!"

Reflecting on the doctor's reply, it was actually refreshing to know that he didn't immediately shun the idea of the energy treatment and alternative therapy. Instead, he marveled over the results.

Again, a helpful aspect of this client's healing was his own level of belief. He believed enough to allow me to work on him and thus, my belief combined with his, certainly raised his overall level of vibration and helped his body to heal itself. What may be news to most, is that as humans on this earth, an energy frequency does indeed run through us. As further proof of a current of energy that constantly runs through us, look no further than the electrocardiogram. What does the electrocardiogram measure? It is a test that helps to determine whether there are problems with the electrical activity or impulses of our hearts.

The final quantifiable proof of this healing of the subject's kidney stone lay within the expertise and indirect endorsement of a modern medical urologist who practices standard, traditional medicine. The stone was gone, and he was without an explanation. I am grateful for this doctor being so forthright.

*   *   *

I believe the kidney stone disintegrated as a result of the combination of powerful focused energy sent into the area, the immense power of visualization, and the build-up of heat over the kidney generated from the energy. With energy healing, the application of the energy can be laser-like when sent into a specified area. I visualized the stone as well as a laser of energy penetrating the center of it, and breaking it up. The client's wish to heal the designated area was also instrumental, for it emitted an energy that collaborated with mine, and formed a strong intention.

We are boundless energetic beings! Many applications have been introduced to us using energy and electricity, especially in recent years with the advancement of technology, but there are even more within the realms of human potential that have still *yet* to be uncovered and revealed. Remember, Energy Healing is a science still in its pioneering stages. It has always existed, but we here in the West are only just discovering it – or catching up to it on a mass level; our collective *conscience* is summoning it! Unfortunately, what we call "science" is a mainstream field comprised of those scientists who only accept something that they can quantifiably measure; that which can be undeniably proven. Tell them about the supernatural or the untapped powers of the mind and the effervescent magnificence of the imagination, and most shall dismiss it with barely a smidgen of consideration, in part due to how they have been trained or programmed, and partly due to the presence of ego and a threat to their own knowledge, and a failure to admit there is much that they do *not* know. This is a mindset that crippled the 20th century, and one that is now being advanced and enlightened.

"Ego" can be a problem when trying to advance something that can benefit all of humanity, and it has negatively reflected upon many men and women who otherwise might have been great, including those industrial barons of the 20th century who stifled the genius of energy giant, Nikola Tesla, because his inventions threatened their profits, power…and egos. Tesla was for the people. He knew about the energy in unseen space. He wanted to give the world free energy and he had the technology to do it. He once lit light bulbs 25 miles away from his lab in Colorado, without the use of wires, and using energy in the unseen he created energetic spectacles over the skies of Long Island. Shutting him down has led to the energy crises we face today – high gas prices, rising electricity costs and utility bills. The truth is that we should only be paying a mere surcharge for all of it – a fraction of what we now pay. Ego, greed and power keeps many in the world in or near poverty. This selfish mindset only harms ourselves and our entire species, stunting growth, evolution and progress, all in exchange for control over the human race and how we live. An estimated 1.5 billion people in this world still do not have access to electricity. Consider that for a moment. If they let Tesla have his way, not only would those barons have solidified their legacies in a more positive light...but also, humanity would be 100 years ahead of where we are now; we would be where we should be, living more selflessly with free energy, less poverty and less war. Instead, we are 100 years behind. Nikola Tesla knew that all of the answers to life and the universe lay in the beautiful and bountiful *unseen* space around us, which directly correlates to the principals of energy healing. According to Tesla, "The day science begins to study non-physical phenomena, it will make more progress in one decade than in all the previous centuries of its existence. To understand the true nature of the universe, one must think in terms of energy, frequency and vibration." This universal and beneficial thinking is long overdue.

PROFILE 3

"I just felt something rise up out of my leg!"
Dealing with Cancer

The events related to this client, occurred early in my energy healing practice. Nonetheless, it remains a memorable experience and the strength of the primary incident has yet to be repeated, at the level it occurred. It is worth discussing at this juncture that just as no two doctors and no two energy healers are the same, similarly, no two people have the same issues, and the pathways to alleviating or releasing them will differ. What I mean by this is that in the realms of energy and energy healing, no two people have the same experiences, blockages and problems that require clearing or healing. A good percentage of these may actually stem from unresolved issues in the past, something that is not frequently considered and thus reveals the varying degrees of complexity that can be involved in the healing process.

Whatever we fail to overcome or learn in our multi-faceted pasts, such as life lessons, only continues to be carried forward, until we face it and/or finally learn from it, subsequently clearing the path, either with the help of others or through working it out ourselves. Revisiting past issues that may have caused trauma, upset or pain can be beneficial in that it can yield answers to current physical or emotional problems. You may find that merely revisiting the past and coming to peace with it, might be enough to bring about a release of a particular issue that you are *currently* experiencing, since the past and the present can be intricately connected. Perhaps you are 'beating yourself up' over a past relationship, or still feeling a deep-rooted guilt from something that happened 20 years ago; both of these examples can manifest physical, bodily issues in the present because they elicit negative, self-defeating emotions and stress. Also, it is uplifting to know that clearing just one thing from our pasts, may clear ten others from our present! It is all connected. It is important to open up those channels that will bring about more awareness of the subtleties still present and still connected to our pasts that may provide further understanding – and hopefully resolve.

Two terms, "opening up" and "awareness" are worth adding to your permanent, mindful list, on which to meditate and focus, because the clues we are given, really can be minutely subtle, and we often need to be consciously awake and in tune with ourselves to recognize them. It is similar to the universe proverbially 'tapping you on the shoulder' to get your attention. You may wake up one day and say to yourself, *I need to make a change in my life,* or after another week at work you may say, *I'm still not feeling fulfilled, and I still feel like I want to do something else with my talents; I'm just not happy.* Often, as I have seen with clients, family and friends, time and again, if we do not acknowledge or respond to the 'shoulder tap' from the universe, we might then be 'pushed' or 'shoved' into a response, which might be in the form of a not-so-pleasant and drastic life event that *forces* us to alter our course; that forces us to act and seek and make a change geared toward more life fulfillment. In these latter instances, there is no choice but to give full attention to the 'life change'.

The subject in this profile, Selma, was diagnosed with the label of non-Hodgkin's lymphoma, prevalent in her right leg. I worked with her following surgery to repair a broken femur, which she sustained as a direct result of the tumor being lodged into the bone, which in turn made the bone unstable; the lymphoma had literally eroded a part of her femur. A titanium rod was inserted into the area to stabilize it, and several rounds of chemotherapy treatments then commenced. I met Selma following some of her chemo treatments, and I quickly discovered that energy healing immediately boosted her vitality and countered the often ill side-effects of the chemotherapy. The side-effects were not as severe following a treatment with me nor did they last as long, compared to their severity and duration *without* an energy treatment.

This finding – effects of energy healing on chemotherapy – came to be recurrent with other clients. I believe this is due to energy healing's ability to work and heal at a cellular level; its ability to bring about rejuvenation of the muscles, organs, blood and cells. In essence, energy healing fosters and aids revitalization, with *no* known negative side-effects.

It was on one particular day when something truly amazing and fascinating occurred, the sort of occurrence that made me fully realize just what the possibilities are with energy healing – they are endless and vast! When I visited Selma, she was experiencing some pain and discomfort, complaining about what felt like a 'kink' over the area where the tumor *was*, and where it intersected with the still fresh titanium rod.

"It just aches right there," she said, some nervousness in her voice, "like something is there. A kink or something."

I immediately began sending energy into the specified area of her leg. Using both hands, I breathed deeply and with each exhale, I sent the whitest light energy I could imagine into her, and when I did, I set the intention to dislodge and release whatever blockage or anomaly was there. When I inhaled, I envisioned the energy literally suctioning the blockage up and *out* of her. As may have already been surmised, setting intentions for a healing is vital when honing in on specific results.

After about thirty minutes into the session, I felt a surge in the energy emitting through my body, through my hands, and into her leg. I felt myself enter into a healing trance, marked by feelings of getting lost in the moment, the healing intention, and the energy that I can often feel pulsating throughout my body; it is an experience of solitude and even bliss. Not soon after, I heard Selma exclaim, "Oh! Oh, my God!" Not a second later, I felt a wave of energy rise up through my hands and seemingly into the air.

"Oh my goodness, did you feel that?" asked Selma.

"Yes, I did."

"I felt it go right up through my leg!"

"And then through my hands. How does your leg feel?" I asked.

She moved her leg and flexed it.

"It's gone. I don't feel any pain or discomfort at all. Whatever was there is gone! The kink is gone," she marveled, her face luminous and bright with joy.

After finishing all of her chemotherapy and radiation treatments, I continued to see Selma for periodic sessions. Eventually, her treatments were no longer for her leg, but rather for relaxation and issues much less in magnitude.

As I type this – three years later – Selma remains healthy and happy, free of the label of cancer.

*   *   *

It is my belief that cancer originates from one of four areas, either singularly or in combination: Life events and stress; environment (natural and/or family, home, work); diets that include an excess of chemicals and non-foods (processed foods), and subliminal awareness of the disease that results in a consistent degree of fear of acquiring the disease. Selma, when she was younger, worked in the medical field as an x-ray technician in the 1950s and early 1960s, where she was exposed to radiation. However, she was also under a rather consistent amount of stress in her home life. Both of these could have contributed to her initial diagnosis. Stress can result in ailments that doctors have difficulty in immediately diagnosing because the origins and early signs of the ailments are usually vague. I have heard client stories, in which their doctors did everything they could to try and pinpoint the root of an ailment in order to treat it, only to come up empty and at a loss for explanation.

Regardless, cancer is a low energy, low frequency disease that carries an equally low vibration, and one's lifestyle *can* play a role. Of course, when it comes to the natural environment – the air, sky, atmosphere – there is little we can do to initially detect poisons and chemicals, but a toxic home or work environment, one that is riddled with negativity, stress, cynicism and/or resentment, can sometimes have equally damaging effects on the human body, and can be just as harmful as chemicals. In fact, chronic stress can have long term effects on the brain, and brain chemistry. Thus, although stress cannot be called a chemical, it can certainly act like one and result in chemical changes in the bodily systems. I further believe that an excess amount of negativity and/or cynicism in one's life can fester and grow into various forms of disease and/or ailments, for it is like poison in the body.

To address the subliminal aspect of disease, which is something I address later in this book, awareness of "cancer" is everywhere in our society. It is in television commercials, fundraisers, ribbons, signage, marathons, and so much more. I believe this all collectively results in the constant presence of both conscious and unconscious fear within the body. This is not good. Society needs to change this dialogue to more positive frequencies.

PROFILE 4

"There is not death. There is only love and life!"

For some first-time clients, energy healing can be an extremely emotional experience, allowing latent or repressed emotions to froth and rise up, often unexpectedly, resulting in a surge of tears and inexplicable crying. This is a cleansing and a release in the rawest of forms, and the most beautiful; a purging of that ever-present issue or issues with which we grew accustomed to living and coexisting. These issues can literally become a part of our subconscious minds after spending so much time weighing down our conscience, and often we acquire the mindset that they are part of us – that as long as we are on this earth, the weighty issues will be with us. However, this does not have to be the case. Following the flow of tears, almost all of my clients react the same way after an unexplained emotional release, uttering the same statement.

"Oh, my God! I don't know where that came from! I was suddenly just overcome..."

Overcome with a significant release of a painful experience or a bundle of cellular memories that – until the healing took place – it was not realized that they had created a neat quagmire in their conscious and emotional state, masked by, or described most often as "numbness", "fogginess", or "heaviness". Does this sound familiar? These experiences or memories are frequently associated with heartache or some form of emotional pain connected to a past event or events that left a lasting impression, and the somber mood associated with the memories always seems close by, coloring your hours and days. If left unchecked it can lead to a depression-like state.

The subject in this profile experienced an emotional release that was connected to the death of a loved one. Roughly midway through our session, he began crying profusely on the table, large, constant tears rolling down his cheeks.

"Oh, I'm so sorry," he said.

"Do not be sorry. There's no reason for you to be," I said, as I went to get him some tissue. "This is good. It is a release. You should feel much lighter after the session is complete."

"I already do. I don't know where this came from."

I smiled. "Yes, you do, and it's been building up over time. Close your eyes. Now take a nice deep breath. Think about the emotion and the tears. *Feel* the emotion. And tell me what the first image is that appears in your mind or the first thought."

The tears flowed again.

"Yes...my Mom. Makes sense. It makes perfect sense."

I continued to work on him, sending in energy. I placed my hands over his heart chakra after first spending time directing energy into his head region, and I visualized holding his heart in my hands and injecting white light energy into it. He immediately breathed an instinctive, full breath of relief.

After the session, I asked what other experiences he might have had.

"I saw some colors flash before my eyes. I could feel the warmth of your hands and...I could sense my Mom."

I told him to drink plenty of water and that the energy from the session would continue to circulate for at least another 48 to 72 hours. The next morning, I received a phone call from him.

"I had a *very* intense dream last night of my Mom. I think I have you to thank for that," he said.

"Thank you for calling and telling me. I am glad to hear that."

"It is a bit of closure for me and it lets me know that she is near. It was really nice seeing her," he said.

"So it was a lucid dream?"

"Yes, I think so. It was very clear. Really nice...and warm. She was right with me, and I guess it was something I needed."

As a society, we have been programmed and told to believe in limits – and in death. The reality is this: There is not death. There is only love and life. We *are* energy. Energy cannot be created or destroyed. Thus, it goes on. I once had a conversation with someone who believed that when we died that was it, the end! I asked her if they could conceive or fathom eternal love, like the love they have for their parents or spouse.

"Yes, I can, but I still believe that when we die, that's it. We're gone."

"Then what?" I asked.

"Then nothing. There's nothing."

"Okay, if you can conceive eternal love and feel it, can you conceive of this nothingness that you speak of?"

"Yes, it's nothing."

"How do you know?" I asked.

She looked at me, "Because I just know."

"How? You just told me there is nothing else. But how do you know what this "nothing" feels like?"

She looked at me in revelation, as if a light bulb had just gone off in her head. She smiled and exclaimed, "Wow! Okay!"

"Okay, what? You said there is just life and it's over, but if there is just life and we're done, then you would not be able to see or sense beyond. You should not and would not have the awareness of another place; another existence. *Nothingness* is every bit a place...and it is every bit an existence, and one that you just now perceived and had the ability to project beyond this physical plane."

She could only continue to smile, mildly bewildered and immersed in deep thought and reflection.

"If that is what you wish to believe," I continued, "so be it. However, I am telling you that that is not the case. There is no such thing as death. It doesn't exist. It is only a notion that we've been trained to believe – like we believe in endings and limits and boundaries. None of this is true. There is only love and life. We transition from one reality to the next. We do not die. Not ever."

*   *   *

In her book, *The Lightworker's Way*, Angelic communicator and Lightworker, Doreen Virtue, confirms the notion that there is only love and life. She recounts the story of how her mother revived her limp and lifeless kitten that had died suddenly. As Doreen recounted:

I remember my mother cradling his limp, lifeless body in her arms as she sat cross-legged on the linoleum kitchen floor. I was crying loudly, begging my mother to do something…My grief was overwhelming, yet I had faith that my mother could save him…As a small child, I had this sort of intense faith in my mother's ability to save my precious little kitten. My mother closed her eyes, and her familiar smile of heavenly love came across her face. She said some commanding words to the cat, such as, "There is no death" and "All is love." Suddenly, I saw movement in the nest of fur. I thought I must be imagining it, yet I also had full faith that my mother's prayers would bring Alfalfa back to me. Sitting about two yards from my mother and Alfalfa, I felt dazed as I watched my kitten come back to life. Where moments before, he'd been limp and lifeless, now he looked like a being thawed from an icy coldness. My mother's expression looked radiant, yet I could see my own surprise reflected in her eyes. She looked dazed, too. I believe that she went into a trance that took her out of normal consciousness. To this day, although she is a lucid and brightly alert person, she only remembers fragments of Alfalfa's healing.[3]

I have often wondered about the expression, 'life after death', and the many people who believe in it, and have had their own experiences. If there is no such thing as death, should the expression then be, 'life after life'? In his 1982 book, *Adventures in Immortality*, George Gallup, Jr. (of *Gallup Poll* fame) explored aspects of this very topic. He surveyed Americans on a variety of immortality and supernatural issues. When he asked Americans, *Do you believe in life after death, or not?* 67% of those polled responded with "YES". Even further, approximately 15 million reported "an other-worldly feeling of union with a divine being."[4] The concept that there is no such thing as death, only love and life, is not new. It has been in our midst for a very long time. According to Robert Lanza, M.D., an advocate of Biocentrism, which espouses that life and consciousness are the keys to the universe, "After the death of his old friend, Albert Einstein said "Now Besso has departed from this strange world a little ahead of me. That means nothing. People like us...know that the distinction between past, present and future is only a stubbornly persistent illusion." New evidence continues to suggest that Einstein was right, death is an illusion."[5] Perhaps society has just been too busy – or too programmed – to notice, or believe. However, I think that having a lack of belief in this concept *could* stifle our own collective power as *ONE*, for it inhibits personal empowerment, forever grasping a finite vision of who we are, rather than an infinite. Remember…energy cannot be destroyed, and we are energy.

PROFILE 5

"For the first time in six or eight months, I
don't have to go to the doctor for an allergy shot!"

There are some occasions when 'on the spot' healings are requested, in locations away from my treatment room. I have discovered that regardless of locale, the energy healing can be just as effective.

The subject in this profile suffered from acute and prolonged allergies that required monthly trips to her doctor, to receive a shot. One day I saw her outside of the confines of my healing room and business. She knew of my practice and had wanted to come see me, but had not yet been able to find the time to do so. When I saw her, she was suffering profusely. Her eyes appeared heavy and tired, and her nose was stuffy, which gave her a nasally voice. She was having difficulty breathing, sleeping and exercising. Her daily life for the past six to eight months or more had become a literal chore as a result of the allergies.

"I so desperately need to come see you. This is just awful," she said, her eyes watering and her cheeks reddened.

"How about right now? Do you have twenty minutes?"

"Yes! Absolutely! I would love it."

We went into an empty room down the hallway. I had her sit comfortably in a standard classroom chair. "Close your eyes and take some nice, deep breaths," I said. "Let yourself go. Think and imagine yourself in a place that will make you very happy; anywhere you want to go. When you feel that happiness, know that this is you *now*! See yourself breathing freely. You *are* breathing freely, without incident or difficulty."

I placed my fingers of one hand on the bridge of her nose, and I placed my other hand on her third eye region *(the chakra and spiritual energy point located in the middle of the brow line). I then began running energy into her. I visualized white light energy to begin. In addition, I initiated deep breathing; to not only raise my own vibration, but hers as well, in the areas of issue.

After about seven or eight minutes, I noted that she was very relaxed. I began visualizing energy flushing the area; back and forth between her third eye region and her entire sinus cavity. By now I had placed my fingers on either side of her nose. I could feel the energy flowing back and forth. I felt my eyes following the energy up and down, as though I was one with it. Since this was my intention, it was thus so – it was happening! Remember, whatever we think about...we bring about!

* The Brow Chakra or 'Third Eye Chakra' is one of 12 known chakras that comprise the system of subtle energy flow throughout our bodies. Together they access a higher mind and spirit. Each individual chakra is a spinning vortex of energy. The word "chakra" comes from the ancient Sanskrit and means "wheel of light." It is pure life force energy. In Energy Healing, they can be used to help bring a body back into balance, for when any one chakra is not operating in its maximum capacity, there is usually imbalance in the particular area associated with that chakra. See *The Complete Guide to Chakras Vintage Edition,* by Ambika Wauters, for more information on chakras.

Following this flushing of energy through the area, what I employed next may sound a bit fanciful and child-like, however, it is every bit imaginative and I can personally attest to its effectiveness with what has become my own style of healing. I began to see myself swimming and/or flying with the energy, flowing with the stream, dousing and sprinkling it through the area. I pictured myself directing large rays or beams of white, gold and indigo-colored energy, into the entire nasal cavity.

"I can see colors," she said, her voice barely audible.

"How do you feel?" I asked.

"Ahh...I feel so relaxed. I feel lighter all over my face."

I resumed my 'swimming and flying' for another five minutes or so, connecting the energy emitted from both hands. I could feel the sides of my own face tingle and my palms buzzing. I then sensed that I should employ something I learned in *Quantum-Touch* Level One. I brought all of the tips of my fingers together, using both hands, forming a more pointed, focused and direct position, like a pirouette. I placed them on either side of her nose and visualized laser-like energy beams coming out of both hand positions – I was aiming for precision. Like a rope tornado or twister I began moving my hands, while in this position, up and down the outer regions of her nasal cavity, cleansing and clearing the areas.

I finished at her head region, directing or 'running energy' into the area, with the intention of clearing and eliminating her stress and exhaustion.

"Oh my God! I feel so much better." She took a deep breath. "It's gone!" She breathed deeply once more. "It's really gone! I can breathe again!"

That night I received a text message from her: *I want you to know that I was able to go to the gym today for the first time in eight months. I was even able to run! Thank you!*

The next day, I received another message from her: *For the first time in six or eight months, I don't have to go to the doctor for an allergy shot!*

In just twenty minutes, something that had riddled this woman's life for months was cleared. Her system became entrained to the healing energy, which created the avenue to heal itself. She remained allergy-free and allergy-shot-free for a whole year, running marathons and taking part in multi-sport events. Only recently did she tell me her allergies had returned, however, they were not as severe as when I had first worked on her; she was no longer incapacitated by them.

Intuition played a major role in this healing. I can definitely feel the intensity of the energy emission continue to grow with every new client and session, and as though in perfect concert and unison, my intuitive skills expand with it. It is as if the energy becomes kindred to me; I become one with it, which only increases the compatibility and the chances for a positive outcome. The overall state of the energy is positive and pure – like love itself!

*   *   *

The reader may ask, *what does it feel like? What does intuition and energy feel like?* I can liken intuition to sensations – *sensing* something within and listening to it; a feeling one gets when they are 'in the zone', focused and attentive – but intuition in this regard can also be a directive, i.e. shift focus to a different area or understanding the origins of an issue. With energy, sometimes I feel as though I can actually touch the energy in the air – or what *appears* to be air. Our ethereal fields and energy signatures can extend several feet outward. Also, like anything, the more something is used or played, i.e. a musical instrument or a sport, the more one acquires a *feel* for that thing. It is no different with sensing and feeling energy, as well as those intuitive messages that come to us daily. Opening up and increasing inner awareness will aid in recognizing the messages so they can benefit you. Learn to have a quiet mind and soul when you need to, as it will amplify your inner gifts, awareness and harmony exponentially. We, as a society, have forgotten what it is like to sit still, in quiet. Yoga and meditation have emerged to help remind us that silence can be a treasured moment of growth. Avoid noisy drama and gossip that steals and drains the *true self*, and that only erodes the quiet within, and ultimately fails to serve us. Engaging in drama and gossip does not equate to meaning, they are temporary and not eternal; they expose the lower, external energies of humanity, and can be an obstacle to inner awareness. Therefore, lessen the drama and increase the meaning. Set aside a part of your day to go within, be wise, speak little, observe...and grow, in stillness! You can begin by noticing and feeling your breath, as it flows inwardly and outwardly through your nose and/or mouth. Focus on nothing else, if but for a few moments every day, and listen within. It is in this way, that I began to develop my own intuition.

PROFILE 6

"I feel so much better, I'm going out dancing!"

In this profile, a "Distant Healing" occurred. What is a Distant Healing? It is a healing done remotely, in this case, over the telephone. I received a text message from Laura, inquiring if I had time to speak with her and conduct a remote session. I called her soon after, and the treatment commenced.

She said she was experiencing joint pain throughout her body and a significant depletion of vitality, to the point of fatigue. Her enthusiasm was on the downswing and she had run out of options on how to rebound, and the frustration was evident in her voice. The client had a previous diagnosis of Lyme disease as well as a significant medical procedure as part of her past medical history.

A Distant Healing is conducted much the same way a physical healing session is conducted, the only obvious difference being the physical presence of the person. However, as I have already intimated earlier in this book, energy hasn't any boundaries, nor does it have any limits. There are some healers I have spoken with, who feel that Distant Healing is even more powerful for them than physical, on-location healing. The manner and techniques I use during a Distant Healing are the same that I use for a physical healing. However, I do accentuate the use of visualization and quantum fields along with the power of my own imagination – I visually image myself being in the room with the subjects, working on them, as if having transported myself there; it can be an extremely sensory experience. It is like playing 'make believe', but it is a completely *real* practice and physical outcome, a true testament to the power of the mind. I have had clients tell me that they can feel *hands* on them or feel sensations in the areas or muscles where I am visualizing and concentrating my presence; where I am placing my hands on them, in my mind and vision. It is an instant assurance and qualified feedback that confirms the power of not only my technique, but the still untapped powers of our minds.

To further illustrate an understanding of Distant Healing for the reader, it is perhaps worthwhile to draw a parallel to the 'identical twin phenomenon'. There have been instances, as you may already know, of one twin experiencing danger or a near-death experience, upon which he/she almost immediately senses and feels the presence of their other half – the other twin. He/she has even reported seeing their identical brother/sister on the scene as a spiritual apparition or spiritual double (similar to 'remote viewing'), as if able to instantly teleport them to the site; or as though their sibling senses that their brother/sister is in trouble and rushes to their side. This clearly illustrates a soulful and spiritual energetic "connection", and perhaps even more, reveals hidden or latent powers within the realms of human potential.

When I spoke to Laura on the phone, I instructed her to sit or lie comfortably. For this session she opted to sit on the floor. I began imagining her as though she was lying on my therapy table, and I was running energy into her temples. I also began visualizing her third eye chakra (located in the middle of the brow line), as I sensed this was a place that needed attention. My intention was to manifest waves of energy going into the areas throughout her forehead region. Laura commented that she could feel *heat* and *tingling* all around her head. Using visualization and intuition, I then began imaging waves of energy literally flushing through her body, from head to toe, back and forth; white and gold energy, with the intention of revitalization and pain removal. She had indicated that the joint pain was centralized chiefly in her shoulder joints and ran down her arms. I soon visualized my hands running energy into first one shoulder, and then the other, deep within, flushing up and down her arms.

I checked in with her to gauge the progress and ascertain if the pain had lessened.

"Yes! I don't feel it in my shoulders and arms anymore, but I feel it in my back and stomach now."

"This is normal," I said, "the pain will sometimes travel."

In *Quantum-Touch*™, it was taught to me as *chasing the pain*. After further study of my own, I came to understand it as an energy block or block of low frequency that is literally dislodged and it seeks or tries to settle elsewhere. I therefore immediately focused my concentration on her abdomen and back, imagining and visualizing my hands sandwiching the area – one hand on her backside, one on her front, over the areas of discomfort, with healthy and positive energy flowing in-between.

It is highly possible to change a low frequency or blocked area, into that of a healthier, high-frequency, free-flowing state. With traveling energy blocks that have been dislodged, I have found that there are two options: To either raise the frequency by injecting more healthy energy thereby dissipating it, or visualize and intend for the block to diminish and rise *out* of the body. I have used both options with success. I typically attempt and use the latter for more serious issues or masses.

After about five more minutes of running energy into the area and chasing the pain, Laura reported that she was entirely pain free. She also reported that she felt relaxed and at ease. Just a couple of hours later, I received a text message from her that read, *Thank you so much! I feel the best I've felt in weeks! I feel so much better I'm going out dancing with my friends!*

*   *   *

Energy knows no distance. It is omnipresent, rotating, circulating, and bountifully available...always. Classic quantum physicists knew this many decades ago, to the point of it being almost elementary in nature. Some may be wondering why these revelations are not taught to our children in schools, or the reader may be asking, *Why am I not aware of this, if this energy is everywhere around me?* I urge you to consider what kind of society or program we have been a part of for the last one hundred years, the factors that control it and those entities that oversee it. I assure you...this energy is real and it is accessible, and *you* can experience it too! I also assure you that our minds have been limited for far too long. Just because you may not have been taught about it…just because you may not be aware of it, does *not* mean it does not exist. We have only scratched the proverbial surface of human potential.

PROFILE 7

Energy Healing Orbs

I have always believed in the existence of orbs, and their representation of the essence of something very special that exists beyond the physical space seen by the naked eye. I believe in that unseen energy, in the unseen space that is in constant, perpetual circulation around us, but as I have already indicated, I have always believed in the possibility of anything. Many people associate orbs with spirits, and while this is true, it must be understood that spirits are energy, and thus, an orb does not always necessarily represent a spirit body; it can be a pure energy perhaps born out of the spiritual – a wondrous, luminous globe that encases all of the love and intention of the healing; a virtual meeting of all things pure, dynamic, untainted, and impeccably immaculate. When the pictures were taken that were connected with this profile, I did not know what to expect – after all, it was not my idea to take the pictures, it was my client's. She had the gifted instinct to try to capture that which she was feeling – the strong circulation of healing energy through her leg.

"I just want to see something," she said, in the midst of our impromptu session that began after I had returned from a gym workout, "I just have a feeling." I was treating Debra because of an injury to her leg. It was an urgent, last minute request due to the severity of the pain she was experiencing.

She was sitting upright, in a chair, and I was seated next to her. Her leg was outstretched, across my knee. She could feel the heat off of my hands, and the pain in her leg was quickly diminishing. That was when she reached for the camera on her phone. She took a few quick photos…and what resulted was awe-inspiring. It was beauty in the form of white light rays and a white energy orb, a perfect and effervescent flow of unison. You can see the photos on my website, where you can see the energy healing orb and rays in all of their splendor, at that amazing moment (www.QuantumEnergyTreatment.com).

One of the slogans of *Quantum-Touch*™ is, "Your Love is Valuable". I display a bumper sticker with the expression that I received from *Quantum-Touch*™, in my office. The meanings behind the slogan are many:

Love is all-powerful; love *can* and *does* heal; one heart emitting love is enough, but many emitting love can save a world. Imagine if every single person in a nation, or in a world emitted pure, heartfelt love all at once? The euphoria would last a century because of the unified, combined heart energy – in fact, we'd probably give birth to a new world. Imagine if we all felt the frequency of love, and always expressed it, saying, "I love you", after we said, "hello" to every person we greeted or met, everyday – imagine what kind of harmonious world we might have. Instead…we as a global society have provided reasons for hate, division and war, stemming from quests for power, money, control, and the passage of laws that only divide us further. My point is that the orb was manifested as a result of the loving core within my intentions – it was an orb created out of universal love and care.

Debra's leg was healed almost instantly, and a black and blue mark from a bruise she had, also disappeared. We waited, after the conclusion the session, for about five minutes, before taking more pictures of the same area, after I had stopped directing and sending energy into Debra's leg. I wanted to ensure that what we had captured was indeed from the energy healing. To my further delight…the orb and rays were gone, without a single trace of them in the photos, which meant they were only present because of the healing energy being emitted/transmitted. It verified the validity of Debra's instinct, sensations and wonderful intuition. It also confirmed that energy healing is indeed a meeting and even a collaboration of client and practitioner/therapist.

*   *   *

When I later reviewed the photos again, I realized that the position of the orb in the photos was exactly the area of Debra's injury; it was the area of primary focus. I intended white light energy into her leg...and a white orb and white light rays appeared; it was a successful manifestation, but one that was initially invisible to the naked eye. I was reminded that Quantum Energy Healing occurs at a molecular level. I thus feel that I can also conclude that the interior of Debra's leg received the same orb and white energy, positively charging muscles, molecules, tendons and cells.

To expound further on how much affect a healer can have on certain conditions, in his book, *Creation of the Universe: Save Yourself*, author Arcady Petrov recounts experiments involving the healer, Oscar Estebany:

In another experiment, the level of hemoglobin was measured in the blood of patients who were being treated by Estebany by the "laying-on of hands." Within a six-day period, the hemoglobin level in these patients increased by an average of 1.2 grams per 100 cubic centimeters of blood. The hemoglobin level of those patients, who refused the services of the healer, did not increase.

Further testing of the water treated by Estebany showed distinct spectrophotometric differences from untreated water. This effect was independently reported by several laboratories. The situation becomes even stranger if we consider the fact that under psychic influence the water molecules became slightly ionized.

This was a serious challenge to conventional physics. The process of transforming atoms and molecules into ions requires substantial energy.[6]

Indeed, substantial energy was evident in the photos with Debra. My session with her was a rare practitioner-client occasion, and one for which I will forever be grateful. One of the most beautiful rewards of becoming a holistic energy practitioner is meeting the wonderful souls who come to me for help. They are seekers of something more; believers in something within, beyond that which we have been taught by schools and mainstream society. In these instances, I become the student, and my clients are the teachers and guides. I learn and grow with them, or rather, I learn and grow *because* of them.

PROFILE 8

*"I feel like the treatments are
taking my mind off it. I feel lighter."*

Thousands of thoughts traverse through our minds daily. For some...those thoughts can be imprisoning. Remember, what we think about, we bring about. This also applies to ailments. It is a good, daily practice to mind your thoughts – pay attention to what you are thinking. Keep them healthy; strive to keep your thoughts good, positive and *in the moment*. Worry and concern only create anxiety and nervousness, sending the body into that dreaded 'fight or flight' mode, taxing the organs and bodily systems further, and yet, so many in our world society are trapped in this brand of existence – always worrying, in 'battle mode', filled with nervous anxiety and ultimately...*controlled* by fear of loss or failure that results in a crippling degree of stress. The body's stressful response may even be powerful enough to either create a new cellular memory or trigger the remembrance of a past memory that was not pleasant, in which your body had to go into protective measure for self-preservation and thus, must do so again because the situation at present is so similar to that one in the past. The patterns repeat and perpetuate, until you resolve to face them, in a disciplined approach, and do something about it – and this could include the cycle of thoughts through your mind.

I fully understand that it is easier "to preach" than "to do", because some circumstances are naturally draining and stressful, and thus unavoidable. However, you must not allow this to be an excuse to not faithfully seek healthier ways. We were not put on this earth to be stressed. We were put here to live, evolve, and be abundant in joy *and* in health! If you can simply increase your awareness of your thoughts, you may be able to combat or eliminate the dreaded worry, concern and stress before it starts, or in the least, make the duration of it under trying conditions, a short one. What are you thinking about right *now*? And how often do you consciously pause to ask yourself this question? Remember…what you think about, you bring about!

The subject in this profile came to the realization that she was thinking and pondering about her condition more than she should. For a long time, she did not realize how much she was fixated on the health issue that seized her mind, which was a bunion on her foot, and it only made the condition more prevalent and pervasive.

Even in the initial consultation I noticed a repetition of questions and concerns.

"Are you sure this is going to work?" she said.

"Let us find out. I am confident we can have a positive effect on it."

"But do you think this energy healing can make it go away?"

"I believe in the possibility of anything," I said. "I know what energy healing can do."

"So you think this can work?"

"Yes, or I would not be an energy healer. I would not be doing this if I did not believe in it. I have a difficult time with insincerity," I said with a laugh.

"But will it take more than one session? Probably, right?"

"I do not know. Some things are fixed in twenty minutes, others over a period of time. It also depends on what *you* believe!" I said with added stress. "If you believe it will take weeks to fix, then it will. Your body and your subconscious mind hear you very well. They also obey you very well."

The exchange gave me an instant, encapsulated view of the mindset of the client. It was obvious that the psyche was playing a major role. In the very first session, I requested that she repeat a series of statements to herself, inaudibly, over and over, feeding suggestions to her conscious and subconscious mind, to begin to reverse belief and thought patterns, while I ran energy into her, with similar intentions.

"I want you to say to yourself, *my body is whole and perfect. I used to have the label of bunion, but it is gone now. It is gone! It is gone! It is gone!* Feel the power of the words. Say them to yourself with conviction and truth! Any past diagnosis is who you *were*, not who you are *now*!"

I sent energy into her temples and forehead for at least half of the hour-long session, and while doing so, I also simultaneously directed an energy flow, in the form of a flush, throughout her body, from her head to her feet.

"Now I want you to take two or three deep breaths, and on your exhale, I want you to image and visualize all of your worries or concerns about anything and everything rise up and *out* of your body. Any and all stress, see it rise up and out, like debris; you are letting it float or fly *away* from you. Then I want you to go to a place that makes you very happy. It can be anywhere you want, but I want you to see it in detail. Once you are there, I want you to see yourself – *feel* yourself – jumping up and down and then running. Look down at your feet and see them perfectly fine; perfectly healthy and whole. See yourself moving in any direction without pain. In this place where you are...there is no such thing as pain or discomfort or stress. It does not exist. And know...this is you *now.*"

I spent the last half of the session sending energy into her heart, solar plexus and her feet. Following the session, I asked what she experienced and how she was feeling.

"My hands were numb about halfway through. My head feels much clearer – almost weightless. I feel good!" she said.

On or about my third session with her, she reported a wonderful revelation. "I feel like the treatments are taking my mind off it," she said. "I feel lighter...mentally lighter. I'm not thinking about the condition as much anymore."

"And are there any concrete results from this?" I asked.

"Yes. I was able to put on my sneakers the other day without even thinking, and there wasn't any pain whatsoever after I tied them up. Everything was fine. I also have more energy. I feel like I have more en-durance."

This further confirmed to me how much influence our minds can have, over not only our bodies, but more specifically, over individual ailments; how it has the power to literally *feed* an ailment. Thus, I reasoned, our minds must then have the same power to *reverse* symptoms stemming from an ailment, if not remove the very ailment itself. After all, it is indeed only a label – it can exist only as much as we allow it to do so.

*   *   *

I believe similar dynamics exist with diseases such as cancer. I believe "we" as an entire global populous of people, or global mind, actually feed and nurture the disease every time we say or read the word! *Cancer* evokes a fright and fear that is difficult to ignore, but it is only a label; it is only a name that someone gave the disease. We ought to change the dialogue and elimi-nate the word from the mainstream so it is not on the tip of our conscience and subconscious mind. Let us demote and disempower the word, and words like it, that only serve to control us and riddle us with fear. It is an example of our fears of a disease literally grow-ing, exacerbating and feeding that disease, which has only made it worse. If we wish to combat and eradicate anything, it begins with shifting our collective focus and de-programming our belief patterns, hence the old adage, *mind over matter*, when "matter" can be "negative or stagnant energy". Rather than having fundraisers and benefits that 'fight cancer', 'run for cancer', 'bike for cancer' or having days dedicated to cancer – all of which are occurring at outrageous levels – change the focus from a negative disease to a positive outcome: Live in *Health*; Run for *Health*; Bike for *Health*; A Day of Living in Perfect *Health* and Harmony! Which one sounds better to you, on which to place your focus? Which is more positive and elicits better feelings in you, the word "cancer" or the word, "health"? The same is true with drug commercials dedicated to the disease. It is all where the focus is placed, for that is where our energy will flow, whether consciously…or unconsciously.

Yes, it is important to get informed about a problem or issue, so you can go about devising a solution. In shifting focus away from the negative I am not advocating to be uninformed about problems, issues and conditions, but rather to use the available information together with your intuition, to positively empower solutions and strategies toward a better outcome. Be aware of the negative influences, but do not allow them to instill fear and/or drown the capacity to see beyond them. The point is to extinguish the negative with a focus on a positive solution, and also the manifestation and awareness of the power that positive energy has over the negative.

The Mayo Clinic's website (mayoclinic.org), has a page dedicated to ways to eliminate or shift negative thinking, and negative thought patterns. Not coincidentally, the page is entitled "Stress Management", and instructs how to practice being positive, and incorporate positive thought into everyday life. As the page concludes, "If you tend to have a negative outlook, don't expect to become an optimist overnight. But with practice, eventually your self-talk will contain less self-criticism and more self-acceptance. You may also become less critical of the world around you. When your state of mind is generally optimistic, you're better able to handle everyday stress in a more constructive way. That ability may contribute to the widely observed health benefits of positive thinking."[7] This demonstrates the Mayo Clinic's – and Western Medicine's – acknowledgement of the influence that mind *can* have over the body and on life.

Unfortunately, on the same page and on the day that I visited the website, there was a Clinic-sponsored banner advertisement for "Killing Cancer". In breaking down the phrase, both of these words are negative and can make the human body stressed and tense by just reading it. This phrase alone directly counters and contradicts the 'positive' information and message on the page. However, it should further demonstrate for the reader the stark contrast and polar opposites that words and phrases can emit. "Killing Cancer" has a negative and very low resonant energetic frequency, while "positive thinking" has a more positive and higher resonant energetic frequency. The point: Always be aware of your thoughts, and the influence that words and phrases have on them. It is all about energy. Words are energy. Thoughts are energy. This is why it is important to 'police' your own mind, and be aware of the information you process. Do not be afraid to ask the question, *what effect is this having on my mind, and on my outlook on life?* It is my belief that negative words and negative thinking alone, can in myriad ways be a formidable disease.

In conclusion, and depending on your habits and daily lifestyles, whether it be a bunion, disease or ailment, taking the master mind *off* the presence of any adverse symptoms experienced and reversing the belief patterns, *can* be powerful enough to remove all of the symptoms entirely! We are *all* healers!

PROFILE 9

"I just felt my neck move!"

Energy healing can be very effective in realigning the bodily structure, i.e. bones, hips, spine. Essentially, what can be achieved with a massage therapist and a chiropractor, can also be achieved through energy healing. It becomes personal preference on what works best for you. However, I will never dissuade anyone from seeking care with another service provider. Not only does it appear manipulative and competitive, but I also feel it is vastly selfish. Wishing success and wellness for everyone, is always a wholesome and positive practice that reaps a higher vibrational frequency, since it emanates from selflessness. I am not only an advocate of other modalities, but I have also been a subject, for not only are there physical benefits derived, but also endless learning experiences that only enhances my own practice, and my ability to help and serve others.

The subject in this healing, Kurt, had been seeing a chiropractor for several years, for recurrent neck and spine issues. He had just begun scheduling sessions with me, as he was seeking an alternative.

"I've just been going for so many years and when I went the other day, it really hurt when my neck was adjusted. I think I now need something less abrupt and forceful."

What I noticed about Kurt was that he made it a point to tell me about every medication he took, accentuating the ailments for which he took them. He seemed to rattle off his ailments and medications as though it was a well-rehearsed monologue; it was obvious he spoke of them often.

Sometimes, when I work with clients, I have found that there are a few minutes at the beginning of the session where I must 'get to know' the energy in particular areas, especially those areas in which there has already been body work or surgery done. The energy will actually feel differently where there was a surgery performed or where there is a blockage, as opposed to chiropractic adjusting or even massage. Every part of the body can also have its own frequency. However, as soon as I began sending energy into Kurt's head region and temples, he drifted off into a trance-like state and I did not feel any energy resistance in the areas. I observed his face and hands twitch repeatedly through-out the first half of the session. About midway through, he emerged from the healing trance and was alert.

"I just felt my neck move! It shifted to the left!" he said.

He had just experienced an adjustment and *release*. I continued working on him, sending energy down his spine and neck. I also urged him to not focus or give attention to any of his *perceived* ailments.

"You are not helping yourself get cured or fixed of the issues that are bothering you by continually talking about them, mentioning them or mindfully fixating on them. Does this make sense?" I said.

"Yes."

"You have just told me about all the things that bother you along with all the medications you are taking. Stop it. It is all connected to *dis-comfort* and *dis-ease*. What you are doing is keeping these health issues ever-present, at the forefront of your conscience. Take your mind off it and your body will respond, and soon follow the suit of your mind."

When he got up off the table, he felt markedly better.

"This was very peaceful," he said. "I could get used to this every day. It didn't have the twists and turns."

He felt like he had gotten aligned without any need for physical manipulation of his bones and joints. Kurt also appeared visibly rested, as though he had just emerged from a long nap. The session was a success.

*   *   *

With regards to the conversation between my client and me, about fixating on the elements connected to his issues, I recall my internship at a rehabilitation and hospice center when I was fulfilling my requirements for *Quantum-Touch™* practitioner certification. It was there where I observed countless numbers of elderly patients and not-so-elderly patients who had simply resigned themselves into sickness or decline. It seemed – perhaps due to lack of attention or love – that they enjoyed talking about all the medications they were on; they also never failed to ask and inquire about when their next medication would be, if they were lucid enough to ask. Whether they craved attention or not, or whether they just wanted to be heard…they had no idea that they were in effect, suppressing their own spirits, miring themselves in unhealthy vibrations, and their bodies were listening – and obeying! It was a self-perpetuating phenomenon. They hadn't the notion that they were only helping to keep themselves in the debil-itated and declining state in which they resided. I will reiterate again, most in our world society do not realize how much power we have over our own bodies, and much of this power is in the most subtle of forms – our thoughts! Collectively, feeding suggestions to our conscious and/or unconscious minds has been making a select number of people in this world very rich! This is one of the main reasons that subliminal advertising has been so successful. What we believe, what we are programmed and *told* to believe…our bodies believe too, and our bodies manifest those beliefs. Do you now see how easy it is for others to profit off of our thoughts? Have you put it all together yet? The energy and frequency to help you awaken to this realization is here now. The maxim is simple: If you want to begin to improve your health, look and go within! As many modern day mystics and thinkers have preached, happiness and health are 'inside' jobs. Avoid discussing your ailments. Do not tell everyone who calls you on the telephone all the medications you might be on – it only helps to keep your body needing them and wanting them. Talk about health and wellness and happiness, not sickness. Our words and thoughts are energetic; they have frequencies…and our bodies mirror these frequencies.

As humans, once we are properly nurtured and matured, it becomes evident that we already have everything we need – food from the earth, wisdom, and the energetic power within, which lead to the faculties to manifest and create *good* things. Learn to be dependent on *you* as much as possible. You *are* powerful, if you *choose* to be.

PROFILE 10

My Travels Through Time

As long as I can recall, I have been fascinated with time travel; its possibilities and its mystique. One of my early attempts at a full-length novel was a time travel love story based in part, on the life of F. Scott Fitzgerald and his unfinished novel, *The Last Tycoon*. I fully immersed myself in research for the book, which included interviews with his authoritative biographer, Matthew Bruccoli – from which a friendship was born – and the study of time travel, quantum physics and the decades in which Scott Fitzgerald lived. Soon after my immersions into this research that only accelerated the fruits of my own imagination, I began having lucid – extremely lucid – time travel dreams. It was almost as if I had put myself into a hypnotic time travel state. I had dipped and coated my entire conscience and sub-conscience into the fanciful, surreal world of another time, and during my nocturnal slumbers, it was all turning over and coming out in full color, the figures and the cities as vital, buoyant and real as the physical reality I knew in my waking state. I was in Times Square, 1920. I felt and saw the bustling city and its people. I recall having the wherewithal in one of those time travel dreams, to grab a newspaper and look at the date. Before my eyes, it went from 1920 to 1998, the dates flipping rapidly as if on a turnstile, the surroundings changing with it. I interacted with some of the people. I saw old trophy cups from a time long past. I ventured into a downtown sidewalk cafe' on a street whose curbs were cleaner than they are today in New York City; I walked past a man reading the newspaper who was wearing a fedora that matched the time. If anyone told me I was not there, I would have said they were lying – this is how *real* it felt to me.

These time travel dreams led me to begin to believe that travels through time just might be possible through hypnosis and/or directly through the *conscious* mind. Ironically, I was reminded of a particular movie and book (both of which I recommend if you like time travel themes) that used hypnotic premises and undertones as devices for time travel: The 1980 film, *Somewhere in Time* and the novel, *Time and Again*, by Jack Finney, which was released in 1970. My dreams occurred in such detail, and they seemed so real, that I kept asking myself, *if we can imagine it, can it be done?* My instinctual answer was – and still is – *yes, I believe so*. Not being an 'official' scientist, I was unable to scientifically confirm or deny my lucid dream experiences. I was also unable to even submit my experiences to any science journals due to lack of 'official' credibility. However, the paradox in all of this is that the field of mainstream science practically refuses to entertain or consider anything born in the imagination or supernatural. It is something, I feel, that has singlehandedly crippled modern science and more specifically, 20th century science, and makes me stop short before regarding it with a complete measure of validity, for I have discovered that the imagination along with that which resides in unseen space – inclusive of the supernatural – is *everything*; it is even where scientific theories are born!

In the field of energy healing...time travel is an application that I have found to be extremely effective. How is this used in the field of energy healing? After being given a set of background and historical facts on the subject, and after determining that some of these are still directly hindering them or are the direct cause of what they are presently experiencing, I will mindfully – using visualization, imagination, and intention –

tap into the subject's past, and travel the tunnel to the episode(s) responsible for the subject's current ailment, illness or adverse condition, to either isolate or neutralize the event(s), or alter its frequency to a more positive state. Most often, these are equivalent to cellular memories; in this case, those highlights of a life that the mind/body has perceptibly classified as "negative", and are wreaking havoc on the subject's current health. The body usually strives to protect us from harmful cellular memories through the 'fight or flight' response, activated by the hypothalamus, but it doesn't erase them or reverse the memories, and the adrenal glands can become stressed in a repetitive 'fight or flight' process, possibly resulting in fatigue, often mistakenly diagnosed as chronic fatigue syndrome, when it actually could be adrenal fatigue.

Earlier in this book, I elaborated on the complexities that can be inherent with health issues; how they can be integrally connected to our past histories. At this juncture, it may be further illuminating to mention that this can also include past lives, which may sound foreign or surprising for those who do not believe in reincarnation. However, remember…energy cannot be destroyed, and we are energy. What might be unresolved or left behind, or what we may fail to grasp or learn in one life, can be carried over to the next life, along with the conditions necessary to finally help us learn and resolve, just like a karmic or soulful balance sheet; the karmic effects of our actions, or what we 'send out'…we get back. It is the constant boomerang effect of life and the soul. I recommend reading Brian Weiss's *Many Masters Many Lives,* and Morey Bernstein's *The Search for Bridey Murphy,* to better understand the subject of past lives, as well the cases of Dr. Jim Tucker, associate professor of psychiatry and neurobehavioral sciences at the University of Virginia, who has researched more than 2,500 children, usually between the ages of 2 and 6 years old, who say they recall a past life. One of Tucker's cases – the case of "Ryan/Marty Martyn" – received nationwide media attention. While it is vitally important to always try to live in the now, it is helpful to know why we might be having the issues and problems we may be contending with in this life, by going *back,* even beyond this life, hence time travel. In energy healing, this outlines the need for the application of time travel, as a tool.

It was the subject in this profile on whom I employed a dose of the time travel technique, in an attempt to lessen the impact of some very painful and disturbing memories that subsequently affected the subject's children and his relationship with them. There had been a very traumatic event that occurred in the early 1960's in which the subject, as an adult, received electric shock treatment therapy, abominably standard for the times. These electric currents administered under stressful and adverse circumstances *do not* leave positive marks and impressions on the psyche. The subject was under medical attention, in some form, for much of the next fifty years, and when I saw him, he appeared to have a lack of mental surety, with occasional fragmentation of thought patterns, especially in verbal expression. Additionally, the subject experienced a childhood with a very dominant parent. There was no overt abuse, but rather high expectations, and what could perhaps be classified as "tough love". Timidity and occasional challenges with self-esteem developed. This pattern was repeated when the subject had children of his own, only it morphed into a passive-aggressive form of occasionally demeaning his children with off-handed comments. This did not reflect the love he had for his children at all – in fact, he was very loving. It was simply how it was all expressed; how *he* was expressed as a result of the litany of trauma and rudimentary procedures that he had experienced and endured. Thus, there were multiple levels of issues that needed attention, love, nurture, resolve...and healing. I sought to peel back the events layer by layer.

When the session began, I started by sending energy into the subject's temples and forehead, while his middle-aged child sat in the room, in a chair adjacent to the table, and looked on. I summoned spirit guides and angels of love and light, and asked for their help in allowing me to be a conduit to the healing. My overall intention was to bring the subject back toward a state of perfection, in body, mind and spirit that brought about some form of reversal for the highest good. With my eyes closed, I visualized traversing through the tunnel that was the subject's life. I sensed some soft blockages at the entrance and cleared those, but I was intent on going back some forty and fifty years, and so I went.

We live and exist in the third dimension. In other dimensions beyond this one, our thoughts manifest instantly. Think *Paris*, you are there. Wish for *New York City, 1975*, and you are there. This is also true in astral travel and astral projection. However, in this profile I was focused on *this* dimension, and traversing the plane of perceptible time. I sped through the tunnel of the subject's life in a matter of seconds and since I knew what kind of blockage there would be, as a result of his traumatic experiences, I was able to sense and recognize the area in that tunnel instantly – it appeared as a very large impediment or mass. I visualized a blast of white light energy at the mass and sent a vibrational tone into it as well, to break it up and raise the vibrational frequency in the area. I then imaged the isolation of the event or mass. The tunnel then cleared. The mass was gone. I then visualized the subject interacting with his child who was in the room with us. I saw the child as a toddler. Once I had the image fixed in my mind, I emitted white and gold light energy into the image, along with a rotating merkaba (two multi-dimensional triangles merged within each other; one upright, the other upside down, also referred to as a spiritual vehicle). Spewing out from the rotating merkaba was still more high-frequency, loving energy that doused the scene and the image. I visualized my hands over his child's heart, sending love and feelings of worthiness, joy and security. It was about that time that I felt something lift – literally lift off the scene, like a cloud of debris. I opened my eyes and saw his child look up at me in surprise, as if something had just happened that was an experience of his own.

"Did you feel anything or have any sensations?" I asked his child immediately after the session completed.

"Yes. It was amazing. That's why I looked at you! I was just sitting there watching you, when I suddenly felt like – like something lifted off my face; my entire being, like a veil or film. It was strange, and after it happened, I felt lighter, more at ease. It's hard to describe."

"I understand," I said. I then explained to him what I had done, using my time travel technique, and how I too had felt something lift.

"Well, I felt it. I mean...something definitely happened and it was just as you looked at me."

As for the subject, he appeared visibly brighter after the session. He felt rejuvenated and spry, although a complete assessment was difficult to discern and ascertain due to the subject's overall state and inability to express himself. While his memories of the events will never be removed and their effects will, in some form, continue to linger, I was content knowing that I had, somehow and in some way, impacted his child in a very positive and enlightening way, using the time travel technique. I also know that on some level, in some layer of the subject's spirit, I had injected a positive, loving influence to counter some of the negative, life-sucking and dark, stressful trauma stemming from the brutal machinations (electric shock therapy) of what was once thought of as 'advanced medicine'. The subject continued periodic sessions. I know that my belief in time travel helped facilitate the event associated with this profile and session.

*   *   *

Zelda Fitzgerald, the wife of F. Scott Fitzgerald, underwent shock therapy treatments during her lifetime. Ironically, her 'before and after' photos are shocking to observe. It appears, in her comparative early life and late life photos, that some vitality and buoyancy of spirit had been drained out of her; out of a woman who was once a beautiful, effervescent and artistic soul – some would even classify her as "brilliant" – only to be reduced and diminished into an abject state. This is not to suggest that there was not a medical condition to be addressed, but rather, to cast light on the brute and unnecessarily harsh treatment prescribed to her that was tragically once deemed part of the new age of medical treatment!

One last thought to consider: If the medical community once thought of shock therapy as 'advanced medicine', why do some in the same medical community outwardly shun, dismiss or reject holistic and alternative therapy? When there is not any blunt and crude alteration of the human physiology and landscape like there was with shock therapy, and even lobotomies? Are the answers only "greed" and "money"? Or is it also "ego" and "ignorance"? After all, in energy healing, there are no pharmaceuticals and medical devices, only pure energy in the form of love and/or wholesome, honest intentions.

PROFILE 11

The Burning Hip

Many times, the cause of an injury is not where the pain is felt. It had been a very harsh winter with one fierce snow storm after another barreling into the East Coast, dumping not inches of the fluffy white stuff – but feet! During the span of one month, there was one wintry storm every week. Needless to say, the winter season quickly turned weary, and the injuries from shoveling snow mounted. The ground was covered with snow for such an extended period of time that even the animals had difficulty foraging for food. Upon the first sign of the spring thaw, people were finally able to breathe a sigh of relief, and tend to their sore bodies.

Jack contacted me to seek remedy for his sore neck and arm, which he blamed on snow shoveling. When he arrived for the session, he described the pain in more detail and in doing so, he inadvertently motioned down along his rib cage, to his right hip.

"Do you know if your hips are aligned?" I asked.

"I doubt they are, especially from the heavy lifting this season," he said.

Standing behind him, and placing two fingers on each hip bone, I was able to eye – or approximately measure – the alignment of his hips. They were way off and out of alignment. His left side was at least two whole inches higher than his right.

One of the first techniques I learned in my *Quantum-Touch*™ workshops was how to realign hips. I immediately administered the technique on Jack, which entailed visualizing and intending the hips to be in perfect balance, and sending energy into both. It can be a fast lesson in the powers of the mind, visualization, intention and manifestation. I sent energy into his hips for a duration of approximately five minutes. When I re-measured their alignment, they were just about level.

"Wow! I can feel that in my legs. It all feels better already," he said.

Once on the treatment table, I focused on his neck and arm, directing white energy into both, amplified by my focused breathing. I have discovered that I have a high success rate in minimizing muscular pain by simply breathing and visualizing white light energy into the muscles. I have noticed that it reduces swelling and almost instantly dissipates the pain, as long as there isn't a more severe injury, such as a muscle or tendon tear, or undetected bone fracture. If the client is not asleep, I will 'check in' with them, to assess their comfort and any sensations during the session. Jack's neck and arm were already feeling better.

I then returned to his right hip, and I 'sandwiched' the location (placing one hand on top/front and one hand on the bottom/back of his hip) and concentrated on sending energy into the area. Jack immediately commented on the intense heat that he felt coming from my hands.

"It's actually burning," he said, "not in a painful way, but more in a healing way."

When energy is flowing the heat will often radiate through my hands. Some clients have even commented that it feels good if they are feeling cold, as if they have a heating pad on them. It is simply the result of concentrated, directed and intended energy flow. When clearings – and healing – occur, it is common to feel such sensations, however feeling sensations or releases are absolutely *not* necessary to experience and receive a healing, or to feel better. Again, everyone is different, with different issues, life paths, and energy signatures, which are likely connected to past histories, life habits, and the choices we inevitably make. Therefore, most every client experiences a different outcome. We are each dynamic in our own unique way.

After the session was over, Jack felt 'lighter', and his body felt better. I advised him to drink plenty of water and to also pay attention to any dreams he might have; we are often given many insights and spiritual messages in our dreams that are intended to help us on our respective life journey. I have discovered that energy healing will occasionally trigger spiritual insights and even visions, stemming from a release or purging that occurred from the healing. Almost always, there is a message to be received in these dreams and visions.

The next day Jack contacted me to tell me, "I don't remember any of my dreams, but I have an overall sense of calm throughout my body. Last night my hips felt like they were on fire. Thanks for a great session – you have great healing hands. Namaste."

Yes, "Namaste"…a divine light is in us all – it is in you. Namaste is the soulful acknowledgement, from one to another; from my heart to yours. I bow to you, my friend.

*   *   *

The realignment of the body is *not* a rare phenomenon in Energy Healing. In fact, Quantum-Touch specifically teaches this as a technique. The movement and shifting of bones occur because the body's structure *wants* to be in alignment, and in perfection. Often times, blockages in other parts of the body may lead to a structure that is out of alignment, perhaps due to compensation from discomfort – favoring one side more than the other. It is something for which the client should troubleshoot and develop an awareness. For instance, a sore foot can lead to a back being out of alignment because the way of walking and standing changes, which puts pressure on the back and causes the posture to change. I have experienced quite a few instances of clients reacting to bodily shifts, after which they feel better, more aligned, lighter, and even more 'grounded', because their structures have returned to their natural and rightful place. When a body is in alignment, energy patterns and chakras become more harmonious throughout the body, organs operate more efficiently and are thus more effective, and the entire system flows as it should. Realignment in Energy Healing is evidence of the power of energy and intention.

PROFILE 12

"I was totally out of my body. I was gone."

The subject in this profile, Cindy, was diagnosed with "chemotherapy resistant" tumors; non-Hodgkin's lymphoma in her chest cavity. One of the two tumors was directly over her heart. Ironically, she had experienced a heartbreaking and psychologically disturbing separation from her spouse, just prior to the diagnosis. Her spiritual seeking later revealed some fascinating and repetitive past life patterns, that *almost* repeated again in this incarnation or life. In other words, she had experienced this pain before, involving the same spouse, in a past life, confirmed by a vivid flashback or vision she had while in the midst of a physical confrontation and life-threatening altercation…when her life literally flashed before her.

Despite the doctor's statement that the malignant tumors were chemotherapy resistant, the physicians still prescribed a full round of chemotherapy and radiation, perhaps in an attempt to halt any *further* spread or formations of the disease. Following a series of three sessions with me – during the same time she was receiving chemotherapy – she went to the doctor for a check-up and PET scan. The scan revealed that the smaller of the two tumors was gone and the larger one, over her heart, had receded and gotten smaller!

"But I'm still not happy," she said to me over the phone. "I wanted them all to be gone. I'm so done with this!"

"You're kidding me!" I said, "The doctors told you these were chemo-resistant, correct?"

"Yes."

"And now you find that one is gone and the other is smaller, right?"

"Yes."

"*That*, is a victory! That's good news! You should be celebrating! The tumors are on their way *out*! To me, it informs us that what we are doing – me and you – is working! Use that positive momentum to your advantage. It should make you breathe a healthy, healing sigh of relief!"

It had been such a grueling experience for her spanning the past twelve months of chemo treatments, doctor visits and mental exhaustion and depletion, that she just wanted it all done. Her attitude during much of the ordeal remained determined and positive – a mental state I believe is essential to counter the disease – in spite of the ever present shock to the human system over having somehow acquired it. The news alone of having the disease is enough to throw the body into instant and constant 'fight or flight' mode.

The doctor's response to the encouraging PET scan results seemed to indicate that they took him by surprise as well: *This is suddenly working; let's keep doing the chemo now.* Thus, another round of chemotherapy was scheduled. I do not think he was really certain exactly *what* was suddenly working. The news pushed her scheduled stem cell treatment back by three months. It also gave me the opportunity to have more sessions with her. During this time, the client was also meeting with a Shamanic practitioner and meditating almost regularly, both of which she had not done before the diagnosis, and that no doubt collectively aided in the healing process. It all led her onto a truly spiritual and beneficial path. I am personally a very big advocate of the Shamans, and I employ some Shamanic techniques into my healing practice.

My next session with the subject was profound. While running energy into her head and chest regions, I felt the presence of something very celestial, even angelic. Midway through the session Cindy entered into a very deep healing trance. Her eyes registered those that might be in a REM state – rolling back and forth, from side to side under closed lids. The energy going into her was extremely strong. She was a unique client in that I could always sense her heart, and this session was no exception; it felt as though her heart was in my hands, receiving all the wonderfully healing, white light energy. I visualized any mass or anomaly rising up and out of her, and taking flight like a flock of butterflies. I also intermittently repeated the following: *It is gone! It is gone! It is gone! Love! Love! Love! Only love resides here!* This was done to counter the negative – if but only perceived – energy of the mass or masses.

In the presence of love and light, there cannot be hate and darkness. Since it was my belief, based on my senses and intuition, that this disease manifested or was attained due to her experiences with impure love and the darkness associated with her former mate, I set my intention to reverse it. This positive reversal would by default rid her body of any physical presence that came about as a result of that previous, past impure love and darkness, essentially undoing it – releasing the negativity from her body. In earlier sessions I had also visualized going back and isolating the figure/spirit responsible for the harm, which I believe laid the groundwork for the gains achieved in future sessions.

When the subject awoke from the session, she reported something that has still, as I write this, not yet been duplicated in detail, vastness and depth.

"I was totally out of my body. I was gone," she said. "I was with a woman with long, flowing hair. I think it was *Mary*. That was who I felt she was...or who I inherently *knew* she was. I also saw you working on me. I saw your energy and aura. But I was with her and we went all over. I felt safe with her."

I worked on the subject several more times and one of most interesting revelations for me, was the literal feeling over her heart, beginning from the first time I worked on her, when the tumor or anomaly was present, in contrast to the last time, when the tumor or anomaly was gone. In that last session, I felt an opening in the area – open space and a flow of life energy that was unimpeded and truly beautiful and free! It became a place where my mind reveled and danced, swirling in that healed area that felt luminous and bright; a field of love, as it should be. I think as her condition improved and her body healed, her mind was also healed, free from the strains of past trauma, like chains, loosened, dropped and disintegrated. She was lighter, in spirit and in body. She was lovely with her power anew, basking in a new light that was all her own...ready to start over, facing life with resplendent vigor. As I write this, Cindy has now been free of cancer and tumors for more than two years, and she has implemented some amazing changes in her life.

PROFILE 13

Menstrual Relief for First Time in Six Months

The physiological mayhem that stress and tense nerves can bring upon a body can be truly confounding – and harmful – resulting in a litany of illnesses and a decline in overall quality of life. When the stress and life pressure is continuous, frequently peppering the bodily system with alarm, forever pressing the internal emergency button (fight or flight response), not only are organs and immune systems affected adversely, but the entire order – the human blueprint – can get disrupted, and its synchronous flow suddenly riddled with irregularity, hindered from the blunt onslaught. In this regard, our systems can metaphorically be likened to machines. The difference is that our oil lubrication and tune up are in the forms of having a more positive outlook and mental state, a less stressful circumstance or condition, and doses of happiness and harmony – those things that make us all pleasantly sigh and take a deep breath of relief. A healthy, balanced, hydrated diet with vital nutrients and proteins can also help.

When the body is in harmony, *not* experiencing stress, all of the systems flow with ease, in perfection; even one's physical appearance improves, the skin breathes easier becoming more vibrant and healthy, and the vital and unimpeded mental state literally reflects in every area of your physical body.

The subject in this profile had the misfortune of experiencing her menstrual cycle non-stop, on a daily, continual basis, for at least six consecutive months. It had been so long that she had forgotten when she *did not* have it. When I saw her, she was under extreme stress and pressure. Mounting family conflicts, the need to earn enough money to survive – which required an adequate job – and going back to school to finish an advanced degree, were all tantamount to the pressures on her mind. She knew what she wanted and what she had to do to get there, but the strains of life were pushing her nerves and body to unhealthy and hazardous limits. She had symptoms of insomnia, sporadic shooting pains across her mid-section and occasional headaches, some bordering on the severity of migraines.

For the first healing session, I planned to concentrate solely on her head region. I wanted her body and mind to once again feel rest, calm and solitude. My first over-all intention was to improve her sleep patterns, which would help her headaches to subside and begin to regulate her system. It is during sleep when our central nervous system is recharged, giving us that sense of re-vitalization upon waking from a deep, restful sleep.

While she did not fall asleep or fall into a healing trance during the first session, she did report the feelings and sensations of heat, tingling and internal movement or shifting. The pulsating pain that she had initially felt in her head, neck and shoulders, began moving and shifting across her chest, toward her stomach. After a few minutes of working on her stomach region...the pain dissipated altogether. After the session, her head felt lighter and her body more relaxed. That night, she slept the longest she had in weeks.

On the second session, which occurred the next day, I shifted my focus to her abdomen and her root and solar plexus chakras. My intention was to restore normal function; to calm the areas and inject some semblance of peace and tranquility in and around the major organs, since they were under great, sustained degrees of stress.

She reported feeling heat, some tingling and, "stuff moving around". I repeated this focus and intention for the next two sessions that followed. All four sessions occurred within a two week period. For some conditions I have discovered that it is very beneficial to conduct the sessions over a very short period of time, building up as much energy in the areas as possible, to counter the severity of the condition.

The day after the fourth session, she told me her menstrual cycle had stopped. She could not recall the last time that her period was *not* an ever-present thought on her mind, for obvious reasons of hygienic and bodily maintenance, and discomfort. There was a slight recurrence of a headache, but it quickly diminished. At times, when areas are healed and cleared, there will be a rise and fall of pain in the same areas of focus. I've come to realize that it is normal following a healing, and liken it to the completion of the purging of the condition(s). Oftentimes, just as fast as the pain or discomfort returns, it subsides. Beyond that of conduction, this is another reason why it is important to drink plenty of water following every session; water helps to flush the areas, and further accentuates the healing.

*   *   *

I did caution her that if she was to continue the stressful habits of her life; those that were toxic and stressful to mind and body, the continual menstruation could very well return. Energy healing may address and/or cure the root of the condition, but if the client fails to alter or change the habits that initially caused it, results will often be temporary.

It is important to pay attention to the trends in your life – and how your body reacts to them. Be aware if you and/or your body feel taxed, fatigued and over-drawn, from the rigors of your lifestyle. If changes are needed for the sake of your well-being, then they need to be made. After all, a body that is unhealthy is never optimally productive. Sometimes in life, we must first make the conscious choice to be well, above all else. Be kind to your body.

My experiences have proven that however difficult or impossible changes in one's life may appear, if per-sistent, continually *seeking* a better quality of life, the opportunity for small, subtle and positive changes will be presented, and like a snowball, the sum of the changes will soon build, and become quite large, re-sulting in a summative impact. You will then likely find life to be quite happier and more harmonious than before. The seeker of good things will always be re-warded, in some way and in some form. If you *really*

want to change your life for the better…you *can*. Remember, we live in a mental, mind-driven universe. We
are all creators. Regardless of your present situation,
believe and *know*…you have more power than you
think you do. If the healings in this book can first be activated and occur through the mind…please consider
the good that you can do with yours. It starts with a
thought and a vision. The goal is happiness.

PROFILE 14

"I always feel better the day after you work on me."

Being a holistic healer does not separate or eliminate the emotional attachment and heartfelt investment that is born out of caring for someone; the same inherent emotions can arise with clients. To be a healer is a belief that there is more that we can do; that we *are* powerful and courageous enough to go within, to heal without. It is a recognition of the ingredients and qualities of human potential that cannot be ignored, but in our largely dependent society, they are often overlooked.

Even in the realm of energy healing there are hearts heavy with empathy, love and constant concern; those clients with whom an emotional or soulful bonding is inevitable. It is like a merging of spirits, in the highest, most intricate, and most sacred of places. Such was the case with the subject of this profile. Her name was

Maxine, and as soon as she became a client, my mission was to save her, and nothing less.

This was a client who came to me as a last resort; a last ditch effort to stave off death. Her cancer was already in the late stages. It had seeped into her bones, liver and pancreas. Most doctors in the western world, upon reading this, would instantly surmise doom and all hope lost. It is one of the stark differences between holistic care and traditional medical care; their guide is what they know and what they have seen. But again, what about that which they do not know? What they have not seen? Those possibilities, however remote, that may never have been discussed in their medical training? How amazing it is to see a person with such a diagnosis *not* give up hope, persevering to the very end – where are the measurements for spirits belonging to these heights? Ask any Western medical doctor about the supernatural or the power of faith, and you will often find that they know less than you do. Yet, there are many stories of people beating and overcoming cancer through faith, diet, will power, and a positive mental attitude, all in conjunction with modern medicine, and it is my belief that these stories will increase, despite what the statistics report, and despite the stark finality given by doctors in their diagnoses.

It was her spouse that had called me first. "Anything you can do! I'm trying everything to save her! Do you think you can do anything?" he said pleadingly.

"I will do everything I can, and I will make myself available as often as you would like," I replied.

The sessions took place at their residence. On the day of the first session, Maxine answered the door after I rang the bell. There I stood, on the doorstep, with my therapy table on my shoulder.

"Yes?" she said. "Are you here for massage or something else?"

"Energy healing. Holistic therapy – "

"Come on in. My husband has called so many people I don't know who is who," she said. "So what do you want me to do? Want me to take off my clothes and get on your table?"

"No!" I said, "No, not at all. Leave your clothes on and get on my table."

"Oh, well that's different," she said.

"I want you to try and relax and lie comfortably," I said. "Take some deep breaths and let yourself sink into the table."

"If I sink into the table will you still find me?" she said with a smile.

After she was on the table I gave her further instructions to begin.

"On your exhales, I want you to imagine all your worries; all your pain and concerns, just floating off you like dust or debris. See it rising off you and drifting away."

"Okay," she said, "my right shoulder really aches right now, if you could do anything for it."

Within just a few moments, after I had begun sending energy into her head, she was fast, fast asleep. I soon felt what I can only describe as a current, one that I had not felt before, flowing or pouring directly into the top-rear of my head, like a channel of constant energy. It was quite amazing to feel and I knew it was going directly into her.

She slept during the entire session. I focused and worked on her head, right shoulder, solar plexus, abdomen and surrounding organs. I visualized sparkling light and set the intention to literally *reverse* damaged cells and *remove* anomalies and impurities; I made it known spiritually that I was open to having it all lift up and out of the subject, using me as a conduit. This does not mean that I 'take on' the issue or ailment. My intentions and the energy flowing through me are wholly positive, trumping by hundreds of times, any negative energy that may be present. Therefore, it is using my positive energy to draw out and replace the negative.

My hands, buzzing with sensations, were swollen and hot with energy flowing through them. I knew that much of it was traversing into her body, as I was still feeling something undeniably physical course through me as well. I visualized the bones of her body being flushed and cleansed with fresh, loving, healing energy.

At the conclusion of the first session, Maxine was a bit groggy. The pain in her shoulder had not dissipated entirely, but it was significantly reduced.

"Yes, it feels better," she said, rotating it.

I suggested another session a couple of days later to fortify and build up her body, before the next chemotherapy treatment that was scheduled for the following week, and they agreed.

By the next day, her overall energy had increased significantly and her appearance, I was told, was more vibrant. She felt good enough for an all-day outing with friends – this for someone diagnosed with the label of late stage cancer.

During the second session the subject again fell into a deep sleep. The same shoulder was still sore although the pains were not as severe as before the first session. I started at her head region, with the intent of raising her vibration to a positive and thus, more powerful state. I then moved to her liver and pancreas and worked on them much more than in the first session, to clear, cleanse and revitalize the organs. I returned to her head region to build up and amplify her mental energies and overall sense of acuity, where I then concluded the session. The chemotherapy regimen she had been through, I knew, was mentally fatiguing and depleting, not to mention the repeated trips to doctors.

I have noticed that when I do work on and around the solar plexus area, I am able to literally flush healing energy from head to toe, like vibratory waves. This is also something I physically *feel* occurring; the energy moving through my hands and upper thorax, pulsing with the waves of energy. For those with the label of "cancer", I have discovered that it is a good way to build up the body before a chemo treatment, to counter the ill-effects. It thus becomes a method of sustenance against the influx of chemicals through the bloodstream, bones and vital organs, complementing all high intentions and for the greatest good.

When she awoke from the second session, she actually looked refreshed. She felt "good" and commented on the warmth emitting from my hands. I also learned that the oncologist had scheduled the subject for a "last ditch effort" experimental chemotherapy cocktail (in addition to the next regular chemotherapy treatment that was part of the most recent 'round'). The so-called *cocktail* was a blend of chemo therapies. I cringed when I heard it, but could only nod my head and listen. It did not sit right with me.

During the routine check-up with the oncologist the next day, in preparation for the regularly scheduled chemotherapy treatment, her oncologist, upon seeing her walk through the door, looked at her and said, "Wow! You look great! What are you doing? Whatever it is, keep it up!" Husband and wife were reluctant at first to divulge *Holistic Therapy*, and only hinted at it, perhaps using the phrase, *Alternative Therapy*. The doctor again said, "Great! Keep it up. The color in your face is amazing."

Following the scheduled chemotherapy treatment, the last in the round before the administration of the experimental cocktail, the subject experienced a worsening of the pain throughout her body and she was exhausted from the ordeal. The side-effects of the chemotherapy had exacerbated everything else, and drained her energy. She requested that I come immediately to work on her.

For this third session, the subject remained awake and alert for the first quarter of it, before falling off into another deep slumber. Before she did, she told me, "I always feel better the day after you work on me." My intention was to "flush and cleanse", which I set about doing. I visualized her organs and aimed to rejuvenate and restore them, reversing any damaged cells. When she awoke at the conclusion of the session, she felt better and I saw that a softness had resurfaced in her eyes. I was glad to see this.

However, something truly miraculous occurred in the time between this third session, and the next time I would see her for the fourth session, separated by a span of four days. When I arrived for the fourth session, her spouse answered the door and ecstatically said, "She's gained seven pounds!"

"Really?" I exclaimed.

"Yes!"

"That's remarkable considering the stage."

"Yes!" he said, "We spent the whole weekend with friends on their boat! She was fine and had a great time! But *seven* pounds!"

I agreed that it was truly a quick and amazing outcome. While Maxine was on the therapy table during this fourth session, she also told me that she wanted to start working out and exercising again.

"I feel really good," she said. "I feel like I want to start going back to the gym or something."

"That's absolutely wonderful," I said. "If that's what you feel, then do it. Start off slowly, using very light weight; even if the workouts are just 15 or 20 minutes to begin."

"Yes, that's what I was thinking. I just have a lot of energy. I feel good."

For the fourth session the intention I set was to thoroughly cleanse the organs and bones *of any and all impurities*, while again flushing and rejuvenating the body. I noticed that Maxine did not sleep during the whole session either, perhaps for only half of it, an indication – I sensed – of the strength and revitalization she was experiencing. Again, she awoke feeling even more refreshed. She was chipper and upbeat, with her natural humor. Before leaving, we scheduled a fifth session.

I again saw her four days later – it was roughly a week and a half before the beginning of follow-up visits and pre-treatment procedures, in preparation for the administration of the experimental chemotherapy cocktail. When I arrived, Maxine was extremely animated – more so than in any prior session. While I worked on her, she shared stories from her childhood which coincided with memories and stories from my own; we even realized that we knew some of the same people. They were poignant, treasured moments that I would not soon forget. It was evident a personal connection had been formed.

I rejuvenated her further. I replenished and I built up her body as much as I humanly and spiritually could, within the range of the abilities and techniques that I knew. It was somewhat hard for me to comprehend that this woman who had gained seven pounds, re-acquired enough vitality to have the desire to exercise again, and who was spending whole weekends out on a boat with friends, was still about to be given a very experimental and thus very risky chemotherapy cocktail. It was not in my authority or place to request another full PET scan first, to see the state of the diagnosed disease in her body; to my knowledge, one was not done while I was treating her, which spanned almost four weeks. At the conclusion of that fifth session, I looked intently into her eyes, shook her hand warmly and left, not knowing what to expect…but I could not ignore the hollow feeling in my gut.

Two and a half weeks went by and I had not heard from Maxine or her spouse. I sent a text message inquiring of the status of her health and the chemotherapy treatment, out of overall concern and curiosity, and as a follow-up. The response that I received left me numb and searching for quite some time: Maxine was indeed given the experimental chemotherapy cocktail, and she was immediately riddled with such severe pain that she was admitted to the hospital, where she quickly succumbed. Her body just couldn't take it, and she passed on, just two days after receiving the cocktail. I could not even bring myself to attend the wake.

I will leave it to the readers to draw their own conclusions as it is not my professional expertise nor my place to even assume a personal conclusion. It has, however, been easy to surmise and make deductions inwardly, based on the facts that I knew regarding her quality of life and state *before* the chemotherapy cocktail. Additionally, any conclusion I might draw could be perceived as tinged with personal affect, as I did attain an attachment to the subject in a very short period of time, partly from my overwhelming desire to help her to heal.

*   *   *

As a healer it was a new experience with new feelings, having an active client expire and transition. It was something with which I had to deal – something unpleasant and unexpected. What does a healer do to heal himself? I allowed the feelings of grief to flow through me, turning over and over like a season, until they became almost malleable and part of my own journey to know myself. In grief, it can be a wise decision to seek to physically *feel* the grieving emotions in order to *release* them that much sooner – to touch them and taste them; it is kindred to getting 'in touch' more with oneself and the myriad of faculties and sensations that traverse through our magical and bountiful spirits. Further, I offered gratitude for the experience, and for the opportunity to work with Maxine; gratitude also for the contrast presented to me, of the extremes, for it aids in the appreciation of the goodness of life. I knew Maxine was in a wonderful place – and I knew I had done all I could; *she* knew I had done all I could.

From time to time, thoughts of Maxine will still pass through my mind. However, I know…there is only love and life, the soul keeps traveling, and it causes me to smile. Across dimensions, spiritual planes, or resplendent fields of pulsating energy, I know that my work with Maxine was not for naught. It is out there, perhaps even spanning across galaxies, my energy with hers, and the immaculate light of her soul.

It is important to remember that we are – each of us – on our own individual journey. When a soul passes on from this plane, the process of passing can be healing for that soul and part of the natural progression, which thus makes it a necessary process. Energy does not remain stagnant. If we are to continue to evolve, we as energetic beings must continue on our path. The torturous aspect can be that we have no way of knowing what the paths of others really are, because it is a relative process – relative to each of us, and of course, there can be heartache over the loss. In this regard, we must simply *trust*. I personally think that this life is like an illusory, holographic playground...and we will all reunite again.

I believe that since each and every one of us will pass on, this mere fact should bind us even closer together. We share a common fate. We will all one day finish and complete our purpose on this plane, and continue to the next. Therefore, this commonality should bring peace, and it should elicit a kinder resolve toward one another, rather than division, conflict or even war. We are transient beings on this earth, mere visitors, fulfilling a journey.

On a final note regarding this profile: Working with any fatal disease requires an abundance of thought and planning. My approach is to go within, carefully ponder the situation, and listen to the guidance of my intuition, before loosely outlining the techniques I will use. I then summon any and all spiritual helpers, and visualize an outcome well in advance of my first session. Occasionally, if I feel it necessary, using visualization I will create a Positive Energy Barrier that emanates and flows out of my crown chakra. I then trust the barrier to serve as my protection.

PROFILE 15

Headaches: A Fast Fix

As a former teacher, I can tell you that very rarely are any two days alike in a public school system. Stressors arise from unseen sources almost daily. In this current U.S. society, the educational system has changed drastically, headlined by the mass attempt to create better test-takers, and *not* individual thinkers who thrive on creativity and imagination, drawing from individual strengths. Teachers are also being subject to increased scrutiny in an observation system that has created countless new judges, many of them ill-prepared to be given such a title, summarily making education more about teachers and systems rather than students and learning. It is not a good recipe. It is also a place (public schools) where not surprisingly, stress-induced ill-health is on the rise, primarily emanating from the hazards associated with mounting pressures and demands. For this reason, the burnout rate in the teaching profession has dramatically risen in recent years.

In the budding days of my healing practice, while I still maintained my position as a special educator in a public high school, I had the opportunity to share my new and emerging holistic energy knowledge, and *Quantum-Touch*™ techniques, with some of my colleagues, one of whom is the subject of this profile. It demonstrates that this work can be done virtually anywhere – including the workplace, where I urge managers and administrators to incorporate on-site holistic healing. Most modalities are non-invasive, quick, easy, and extremely beneficial, bringing about at least some degree of instant relief.

Elijah had been experiencing severe headaches for several days, and he was also feeling stiffness and discomfort across his shoulder blades. All of it, I knew and sensed, was stress-related. Coupled with a hectic family life, the pressures from the implementation of the new observational system added more stress and compounded existing strains. The psychological stress from not knowing exactly when someone might come into the classroom to essentially observe and grade his performance, perhaps taking entire moments out of context if in the midst of a lesson, were wreaking havoc on the mind of not only this teacher, but also on those throughout the school; teaching suddenly seemed like a never-ending audition, teaching pre-set and pre-determined material in ways and methods that were also pre-determined, much like a robot or automaton, regardless of individual student strengths or weaknesses. Paranoia had slowly pervaded the teaching atmosphere, and children, as sharp and acute of mind as they can be, also sensed this.

I told Elijah I could probably help him during my lunch period, for about 15 minutes. He was desperate for a solution.

"I'll try anything. I took some over-the-counter pain medicine, but it's not working. The pain is shooting across my forehead and I can feel it building," he said.

We met in my room, and I had him sit in a standard classroom chair. I stood behind him, placed my hands on either side of his forehead, and began sending energy into him. I told him to close his eyes and relax as best he could. I also instructed him to visualize a place of peace and love; to imagine he was there and to see it in as much detail as possible.

"In this place," I continued, "there is not any such thing as stress or pressure. There is only love and harmony. Feel this. Perhaps you are on a beach or in a green field. Look down and imagine that you see your feet firmly planted. Feel the joy and happiness of the experience."

Elijah quickly approached the beginnings of a healing trance; he was suddenly extremely relaxed and drifting in and out of REM state. To add to the stress he had been experiencing, by default, he was also feeling fatigued. I began swirling the energy to and fro, between my hands, flushing his entire frontal lobe area. I sent the energy, through intention, down into his eyes. I could feel the heat coming off my hands and noted the swelling of my fingers from the energy rushing through them.

After I sent energy into his head region, I moved my hands to his shoulders, which were extremely tight and tense. I placed both hands flush against him, but without applying pressure. I then sent/intended white and gold energy into his upper back, shoulders and neck. Within only a few moments, I could quickly feel some of the stiffness dissipate and his muscles release.

After about 15 minutes, with my hands still on his shoulders, I told him to slowly open his eyes.

"How do you feel?"

"Wow! I feel so much more rested."

"How does your head feel?" I asked.

"Much better," he said. He turned his head from side to side. "The pain is gone. My shoulders feel better too. That's amazing. I feel like I could go to sleep I'm so relaxed."

I told him to make sure he got a bottle of water, and I instructed him to sip it for the rest of the day, and to also drink more water later that evening. It was an almost instantaneous fix for his ailments and it remained that way for at least a month. Since he remained in his education position, and his schedule and the demands on him did not change, naturally, some pain and discomfort did eventually return, however, it was evidence that energy healing was a viable treatment alternative, indicated by the results. In fact, for a time, he would periodically inquire about my practice and recall the wonderful experience he had.

"It's amazing. I believe in what you do." he said.

I feel that very soon, as the awareness of holistic energy healing as a remedy circulates and grows, many more people will believe in it as well. It brought me great joy and satisfaction that I could help him through some difficult times and cope with an incredibly stressful situation. Again, this profile demonstrates holistic energy healing as an asset in the workplace. In this time of spiking healthcare costs, its value as a preventative therapy could be immeasurable.

PROFILE 16

Structural Realignment from a Car Accident

The subject in this profile experienced a car accident roughly eight months before I saw her as a client. The impact was so severe that it significantly shifted her neck and spine toward her left shoulder. As a result of the injury, painful headaches, backaches and muscle aches became the norm. Her job, which necessitated her to carry a backpack as her briefcase, only exacerbated the issues, and strained her body further. The subject was also seeing a chiropractor and she had personally ruled out surgery, opting to care for her issue naturally and holistically. She felt and perceived that the option of surgery presented too much of a risk and would threaten her quality of life even further, since it would involve an operation on her spine and spinal region. She was very much in touch with her body and possessed a strong self-awareness, and thus, she felt more than comfortable assessing herself and making this decision on her own volition.

When administering care to clients with these types of cases and/or issues stemming from an accident, I have found that it is important to set the intentions for the session in a high vibrational resonance; words and images that are absolutely positive and that naturally elicit positive feelings and emotions. If I set such intentions, it is by default that when I see the images associated with them in my mind, I will experience and *feel* emotions of love and positivity, all high in frequency and thus vibration. When I feel this, my client will as well, and the area will be injected and doused with this higher vibration which will aid in healing the area, entraining her energy to the positive intentions. Remember, injuries are areas of low vibrational frequency, and it is always the aim of the healer to raise the vibration in these areas.

I focused the entire session on her head, neck, shoulder and upper back regions, with the brunt of the session on C1 through C7 of her cervical vertebrae. I visualized the subject moving freely, without pain and hindrance, smiling and happy, and I set this as my overall intention; this also an attempt to elicit a shapeshift in the physical domain through accessing the spiritual body blueprint, in which we are *all* per-

fect. I then set a secondary intention, likened to bench-
marks or individual objectives to accomplish in route
to the overarching primary intention: *To shift her vertebrae and spinal column back into original wholeness and
perfection.*

During the session, she commented that she could
feel intense heat in the focused areas. She did not fall
asleep and remained alert throughout. I began volley-
ing the energy like a ping pong ball, back and forth between my hands, which were placed on either side of
her head, before moving my hands to her neck. There
was an instance or two when she said that she felt pain
moving down toward her shoulders, and in these instances, I "chased the pain", tracked it and dissolved it,
then returned to her neck and head as targeted regions,
while carefully listening to my intuitions.

It is worth noting here that after the intentions are
set and established, it is not necessary to fixate or return to them mindfully, and certainly not what might
be deemed "obsessively". As a healer, I set them and
forget them, trusting they have been set into motion by
my thoughts alone, which again, are pure energy. As
soon as I "think" the intentions, energy and molecules
are set into motion. Unless intuition tells me to focus
on them again, or change them to something else, I

leave them in trust and love and move my attention to the energy itself.

Roughly three-quarters through the session, the subject suddenly exclaimed, "Something just moved. It shifted."

"Where did you feel it?" I asked.

"Right in my neck, it's like it just moved into alignment like I experience at the chiropractor's, but this was a bit different because you didn't jerk my neck and the whole area moved."

"You are not in any pain are you?"

"No, not at all."

Suffice to say, the subject did experience a re-alignment. The next day her neck muscles and upper back muscles surrounding her spine were very sore. "Like a good soreness," she reported. It made perfect sense that she would be sore since the muscles were re-acclimating to the re-alignment, compensating for the movement back into wholeness.

* * *

Unfortunately, the subject also returned to work the next day – back to bodily and mental stress; she returned to the very routine that had become a habitual part of her life. Even though she sustained her injuries in a car accident, the demands of her job re-aggravated the injuries, and it wasn't long after when she required more adjusting, and more body work. As seen in a previous case profile, such toxic and stressful lifestyles wreak perpetual havoc on the body, and eventually, the mind. Aside from the spells of relief that will be experienced, achieving a permanent healing can be difficult in these situations. My advice: Seek a career or job that does not present so much stress. Life is far too short to bask in misery – unless you are the sort that thrives on stress, but even still, the body can only take so much. I realize economic or family situations and demands may not be optimum for such a switch, and if so, then I recommend that you hold in your mind the kind of job and life that you *do* want. See it. Visualize it in every detail you can imagine. It should be a fun process, without force or effort, as if you are on a mindful holiday to the reality of your heart's highest aspirations. It should create positive, happy feelings in you.

Forming the discipline to focus on, and see what you desire, on a daily basis, if but for just five minutes each time, can be a form of extremely beneficial meditation, and you may find that you want to do it more often, which is perfectly fine, but what it also does, like intentions, is it puts energy and molecules into motion. Perhaps not the next day or the next month, or even the next year, but soon, you will start to notice a better disposition and mood; you may notice that what bothered you constantly, does not bother you so much anymore, replaced by a more positive outlook. You will start to *notice* more often; noticing the nuances and fine aspects of life to which you may not have previously had the mind and awareness to even pay attention. You may also notice more opportunities coming your way and into your life, such as job prospects, ideas or resolutions. I urge you to *see* the ultimate reality you want to create. Then, do not worry about how it will happen...just trust and leave it all to the universe! The new age into which mankind is entering will see our thoughts manifest and come to fruition faster than ever before – in other words, you may find that your thoughts will come true or manifest into your reality as something "real", much faster. So...why not start having fun with it now – you never know what you might create for yourself. The age-old adage, *be careful what you wish for, you just might get it*, will never be more true and have more resonance, than in this amazing golden age into which we are all slowly entering.

PROFILE 17

"My lungs are definitely not as congested."

Keith, the subject in this *distant healing* profile, was experiencing severe congestion in his lung and chest cavities stemming from fungal growth, the cumulative result of chronic asthma and allergies. He was having tremendous difficulty breathing, each breath intensely labored and audible, inclusive of when he spoke. He would often have to pause mid-sentence and digress into a long, wheezing cough, accentuated by his efforts to clear the blockages and congestion. The area where he lived was also a contributor to his ailments – the oft dusty confines of Midwestern America. He had been seeking care from a naturopath and chiropractor. Depleted finances and lack of adequate healthcare coverage prevented him from going to his traditional primary care physician; however, this traditional route had previously been unsuccessful in relieving the symptoms and eliminating the condition, and thus, it was actually a non-issue for him.

For this healing, I informed Keith that I would be working on him after we ended the phone call and disconnected. I advised him to sit comfortably on his couch for the next 30 minutes, and simply pay attention to anything he might feel. I also cautioned him not to be *expecting* anything, but simply be *open* to receiving.

When I commenced the session, I was careful not to force anything; not to forcefully push or "blast" the energy into him, but rather let it slowly build and evolve based on what I sensed from afar, in accordance to my visualizations. I wanted the energy to gently circulate, dissolving and/or replacing the fungus, and essentially 'unclogging' the area(s). I also did not start at his head region, but rather went directly to each side of his rib/lung areas, where I immediately began injecting energy and intention, just as I would in a physical, on-site session.

With my eyes closed and seated comfortably on my own couch, I visualized my hands on the areas of issue, emitting a white, healthy energy that his lung and chest regions readily absorbed. My intention was to *clear* the areas and bring immediate relief of his symptoms. I began alternating my visions between sending energy into him, to seeing him breathe without effort; joyous and smiling, in perfect health. About midway through the session, through visualization, I moved my hands to his chest region, where I resumed my energy emissions.

After roughly thirty minutes of distant healing, I telephoned Keith and inquired how he felt.

"I felt heat in my ribs, lung and chest areas."

"How is your breathing?" I asked.

"My lungs are definitely not as congested. I'd say my breathing is about 40% better."

"Very good –"

"Yeah, it definitely worked."

*   *   *

It has been said that life is a hologram, an illusion of our own creation, and energy – like our thoughts of another in a faraway place – knows no distance. It is worthy to note to the reader, if not understood already, that the act of visualizing can be exactly the same as being with the subject in person. Yes, *belief* does play a role. However, what one knows through experience, one then believes. What I have come to conclude through my experiences, going back to when I was a child and also through the use of my creative imagination, is that the power of the mind is far more powerful than what we are taught, and it is more powerful than what is espoused in the mainstream – I *believe* in the power of my mind, and *you* should believe in the power of yours. I have experienced absolute results through its use; through visualization and implementing the vast faculties of my imagination. I inherently know it is all very real and it is very true, and recent discoveries in quantum mechanics and quantum physics support these beliefs. While these experiences may be relative to me, they can be effective and *can work for you as well*. It starts with belief in that which you do not know; in the unseen. Many holy books even stress the powers of belief and positive intentions, and the amazing results that can occur, sometimes called "miracles". I urge you all to explore your own minds and beliefs like a child. As an exercise, take five idle minutes and daydream like you never have – or in a way that you have not done since you were a child. Explore the *what ifs*, and marvel at what your imagination concocts. To fantasize is valuable, because it is giving your imagination a workout – it is our own virtual reality console, and it can also be a stress reliever. Even more, try to fantasize with an intention to manifest, for it then directly correlates with intended visualization.

What we have been taught and told and pro-grammed to believe by our society, is indeed equiva-lent to still harboring the mindset of an infant. For what do we really know except that which we have been told? How much of your respective lives is a re-sult of your *own* discoveries? Or are you living accord-ing to someone else's discoveries? But even more…how do we know that all we have been told is true; that it is *our* truth and more importantly, *your* truth?

Believe more often. Seek new ways to live, witness and experience your reality. Reactivate and become fa-miliar – or more familiar – with your imagination, and imagine for yourselves, seeing and realizing the greater, boundless frontiers that can emerge and that await you, ones that *are* attainable – they always have been, and then prepare to be enlightened, and enlight-enment will be yours, relative to *you*. Visualization is only a small particle of the still untapped, ever-abounding existence within us all that has the potential to bloom and literally become us. It is part of recon-necting with who we are; reconnecting with our very existence! *Believe. Imagine. Empower* yourselves…and awaken! What you see in your mind can be your real-ity…it *is* your reality, and you do not need anyone to tell you so. You are limitless.

PROFILE 18

Taking Inches Off the Waist

The client in this profile, Cynthia, came to me seeking a cure for the diastasis she had developed following her last pregnancy. Diastasis is a widening of the belly muscles, also referred to as "abdominal separation". It is quite common for women to acquire diastasis if they have been pregnant more than once. Pregnancy results in so much pressure on the abdominal muscles that sometimes they just cannot maintain their shape, hence the condition. The muscles often need to be retrained and tightened to regain their shape, and realign. Doctors will occasionally recommend a belly splint to hold and/or bring the abdominal muscles back together. With diastasis, a healing of the overstretched abdominal muscles is needed.

Cynthia had been prescribed abdominal exercises by her doctor, as a remedy for the diastasis. However, she wanted another alternative because she did not feel the exercises were completely effective. Her aim was to decrease her waistline by at least a couple of inches.

Energy healing, I have discovered, increases the flow of everything in the areas of focus; it increases circulation, oxygen, molecular movement...and energy. When intending or running energy into a particular area, I can often feel a rise of activity in that area. One way I can attempt to describe it is through the idea that rubbing coffee grinds on waistlines decreases cellulite. It has, for years, been a common trick used by many beauty models. Coffee is a stimulant that 'stimulates' the surface area on the waist. Likewise, energy healing stimulates activity within and throughout the body, activating the body's own ability to return to wholeness and perfection.

The first time I saw Cynthia for a session, was the day before she was to see her doctor. She admitted that she hadn't been doing the prescribed exercises as frequently as she should. I ran energy into her abdominal cavity and on either side of her waistline. I could feel the energy pulsating back and forth, and I could also feel it through my hands. The session went smoothly and the next day, Cynthia went to see her doctor.

"My doctor told me I looked good and to keep doing the exercises," said Cynthia.

She scheduled a second session a couple of weeks later. This time she admitted that she had not been doing the exercises at all.

"I just feel really good and I think the last session helped. I'm not going to tell my doctor I haven't been doing the exercises though!" she said with a laugh.

Once again, I ran energy into her, focusing primarily on her upper and lower abdominal areas and waistline. I recall being fascinated with the contrast of sensations in the area, between the first session and the second session. Her abdominal area felt different; it felt healthier with fewer blockages than in the first session. The energy seemed to flow better than before. I have come to detect such differences simply through repeated sessions with clients – through my collective experience. The areas of focus will not feel as 'thick' or 'dense', and the energy will flow without impediment. Again, as I've already alluded, if you work with energy enough, an element of intuition develops. It is intuition, inner awareness, focus, and 'tuning in' to the client that can elicit the identification of such differences, and associated improvements.

A couple of weeks later, after her follow-up visit with her doctor, Cynthia sent me a text message: *I lost probably four inches off my waist. The doctor said the exer-*

cises were working. I didn't tell her that I hadn't been doing them!

Cynthia did not feel the need to see me again for this condition. Subsequent sessions were for issues completely unrelated – and her waistline was back into shape.

*   *   *

Following every full energy session, the energy will continue to circulate and 'work', for up to 72 hours. Therefore, the benefits continue long after the conclusion of the session. I will frankly admit that I was not expecting such a drastic reduction in Cynthia's waistline, but I was certainly *intending* perfection and wholeness in the area. Energy is intelligent. It is source energy. It goes where it needs to go. This is one of the reasons I am forever fascinated with energy healing – the results can be absolutely extraordinary, and I often marvel in wonder over the prospect of its untapped, endless potential. It is my belief that the two energy sessions accelerated the healing of Cynthia's abdominal muscles; it activated and stimulated them back into harmony. Also, it cannot be overlooked that Cynthia knew what she needed, hence another instance of the combined intentions of client and practitioner.

This profile further demonstrates the myriad of applications for energy healing; in fact, the potential applications are countless. In an hour-long interview I did with *Quantum-Touch*™ founder, Richard Gordon, we discussed the unlimited applications of energy healing, along with some of the profiles featured in this book. The interview can be found on *YouTube*, in the *Quantum-Touch*™ channel, or by searching my name.

What You Can Do –
We Are All Healers

1. **Pause. Notice. Reflect.** In the midst of your day, at any given, unplanned moment – *pause*. Look around you. Notice the colors, the people and any objects. Try to sense the pulse of the world that you are in. Reflect on any meaning that comes to you; the subtle messages that your intuition may be providing. Breathe easy. Offer gratitude. And smile. It is most often in stillness and observation when we are moved…and when we grow.

2. **Be in the moment. Ask yourself,** *what am I doing now?* The question will help you to stay in the moment. It is vitally important to be in the present, for that is the only moment we have to work with. As a healer, being in the moment aids the intuition; it leads to becoming an active, more attentive listener, within *and* without. In our present high-tech society,

proper listening is now a skill to master. Being in the moment also keeps you out of your head – it is a surefire way to discipline the mind and keep it from wandering to gossip, past troubles, and future worries. Discipline yourself to stay in the *now*.

3. **Take a quiet moment to think of something or someone that brings love to your heart.** Feel the love. Think about the love. Your moment will be flooded with that beautiful healing love, and it will not only affect you, but perhaps those around you and the immediate space or room where you are reflecting, because it is such a powerful energetic emotion. Remember, love is healing and all powerful. Once you feel the love…take a deep, easy inhale, then exhale with peace and harmony through your heart and/or heart chakra – breathe out through your heart, get in tune with its magnificence, and feel your heart energy. This can be a very meditative and euphoric experience; it can quickly eliminate stress and bring solitude.

4. **Offer gratitude in large, constant doses – for everything! And do it with a smile.** Gratitude is power, and it can quickly put you in a state of high vibration and resonance – optimum healing states for you and others. You can start with something

like this: *Thank you so much for me! Thank you for this day, my health, my food, my shelter, my love; thank you for the way I view the world, for I am grateful. Thank you for all of my experiences, good and bad, for they teach me to know the difference between extremes. Thank you for now!* Every day when I wake up I say, "thank you." And almost every morning when I come down my stairs to make my coffee I say, "thank you," on every step I descend. It is a great, positive and powerful way to start your day. *Thank you! Thank you! Thank you!* Whenever I remember, I will even thank the water I drink.

5. **Place your open hands flat, flush against both sides of your stomach or abdomen.** Take an easy, deep breath in…and out. When you breathe in and out again, on your exhale, envision any worries, concerns or needless thoughts floating up and away like butterflies – the more detail you can give your butterflies, the more it will draw you in, to the serenity of the vision. What is the design on their wings? Stay in the moment of breathing. Feel your breath. Listen to your resplendent heartbeat. Now slowly breathe in again…and when you breathe out, close your eyes and breathe through your hands, and envision white light energy going through your hands and into

your stomach/abdomen or solar plexus region. Repeat until you begin to feel the increased warmth of your hands on your skin. Do not force the breath, but allow the whole exercise to flow with ease, joy, trust and peace. The exercise can quickly bring moments of peace and tranquility; a mindful vacation that is a form of self-healing.

6. **Lay your hands on a loved one. It can also be a pet if you choose.** Feel the exchange of warmth, love and *being*. Breathe through your hands. Breathe love from your heart. Envision a color for your heart energy and breathe it into your loved one, see the color absorbing. Lay in silence and listen to each other's breathing – you may find, by the end of this exercise that you are both breathing at the same tempo, in unison and entrainment. Continue to be in the moment, and what a beautiful, harmonious moment it shall be. If you are not used to doing exercises of this nature with your partner, there may be discomfort or uncomfortable laughter in the first few moments or attempts, but it will eventually subside. Do this until there is a mutual sense of peace and calm, within and without. You may even feel or sense a bonding as *One*. This is also an excellent exercise to

surpass disagreement or discord. Again, just trust the process, surrender, and enjoy.

7. **Visualize.** It has been my experience that visualization in the healing arts is one of the most powerful processes to undertake. I believe visualization is a combination of imagination and belief, which, as a friend of mine pointed out, according to this definition "it is the opposite of worry." Dare to imagine beyond your normal boundaries...then dare to believe in it all. The process will also naturally elicit feelings associated and connected with your visualizations; emotions that serve to charge the visualizations and even the outcome. When I work with clients and employ visualization, I will visualize with detail going *into* the area of issue; *into* the muscles, *into* the bones, or *into* blood streams, sending and intending energy and love to the places of need. To illustrate the power of visualization, sit calmly and comfortably on a sofa or chair, and close your eyes. Visualize that you are doing sit-ups, push-ups or an exercise of your choice. See yourself in detail – in your mind – actually doing the exercise. You should be able to see and describe the locale, the athletic shoes on your feet, and perhaps even what you are wearing. Do this for at least a few minutes *with-*

out strain. Concentrate, and keep doing the exercise only *in your mind*, until you feel it. What do you feel in your body? Are the muscles associated with that given exercise getting warm? Twitching? Jerking? If so, this is because your muscles don't know the difference between doing the exercise and not doing the exercise – but it does receive the messages that you are sending in your mind. Your muscles and bones know the parts that need to be used in order to complete your visualized exercise. Yes, this means you could theoretically do an entire gym workout in your mind – and your muscles will *feel* it! Again, this should be an enjoyable and fun exercise, and not one of labor. Think about what this could mean for healing. Therefore, have fun and experiment! Visualize white and gold energy being sent to areas of your body that may be in need....visualize sending energy to others, with the energy dancing, soaking and absorbing into your intended areas – and healing. Then finish with the mantra, *it is thus so, so be it!*

8. **Create a healthy, positively-charged environment.** Too often, people exist in very negative environments, whether it be in their home, their workplace, and/or anywhere they may spend a large amount of time. This can be extremely draining on

the body and mind; it can feel smothering because negative energy is often pervasive. It is important to be mindful and aware of the energies in which you reside. If the energies feel negative and/or stale, try to change them, whether that be through smudging with sage and sweetgrass, using incense, opening a window, listening to pleasant music, or hanging a beautiful picture on the wall that moves you to visualize equally beautiful imagery; do something healthy in that environment that makes you feel good. You can also change how you interact with that environment, and it starts with your thoughts – you have the power to impact any environment with your thoughts alone. If you live or work with someone who is overtly negative and who adversely affects the environment, be sure you don't *digest* all of their negativity and disempowering words. Immediately dismiss the negative aspects in your mind, and project the environment that you would like to have. At work, put on your headphones if you are allowed, and listen to that pleasant music. At home, perhaps try to set up boundaries for what is designated as *your space* and/or *your time*, in which to meditate or bask in your own peace. *Intend* to make your environment positive, peaceful and happy, and do what you can to make it so. It can be a relief to remember that positive energy is hundreds of times more powerful than negative energy.

9. **Do your part.** This is the Age of Healing, a time when the magnitude of our true selves – our human potential – is just starting to be realized. Do your part to read, study, and research other methodologies and modes of healing; explore other possible ways toward better health and well-being – I have provided one possibility in this book. Analyze and examine new breakthroughs in medical science that are not being reported in the mainstream. Be an independent thinker and self-advocate for your health, rather than automatically accepting those ways, procedures and regimens that are *told to you*. Be proactive. Ask questions! Ask, *why?* And sometimes, be willing to challenge the supposed authority of others. Just because they have a title, does not always make them smarter than you. The United States now has a different healthcare system under the Affordable Care Act. I have a family member who went to see three different doctors for a condition. All three recommended a PET scan. However, since the passage of the Affordable Care Act, there is now a 'ruling authority' (also known as a benefits management company) who determines whether a procedure is

necessary, and thus whether respective insurance companies should pay for it; they are in place to "lower costs" and save insurance companies money. Should it then be reasoned that they consider 'cost saving' before they consider 'human life'? Members of this ruling authority never met the family member who had the condition; no one on the board ever saw them as a patient, and yet, they promptly *over-ruled* all three of their doctors, and *denied* the PET scan. What does this mean? It means the sanctity of human life is being thrown into the balance. If situations like this persist, Western medicine risks losing a significant amount of relevance – and quality of healthcare. As stated at the beginning of this book, medical error is the third leading cause of death in the United States. With a ruling authority such as this, should we expect this statistic to increase or diminish? Bottom line: Do your part to take control of your own healing. Be informed. Be knowledgeable. Work *with* your doctor(s) to arrive at the best approach for given conditions, and do not be afraid to broach the subject of alternative healing as a complementary modality.

Post Commentary and Thoughts

Spiritual awakening is something that must come from within. It is not something one simply wakes up to, but rather, something one seeks and aspires to attain, and/or to experience. It is, from my own experiences, one of the most beautiful of things to be sought. It is like a brush of Heaven while planted on earth. Once attained, it is something from which to constantly draw; for strength, for base and foundation. Spiritual awakening is a state of being that, depending on one's life and the circumstances that might arise, can come and go. However, once you know what it feels like, should life veer off course, however temporary, it is a place to return to, and find refuge. You come to know it, like a dear friend – or rather, your dear soul. Spiritual awakening is a slice of euphoria that colors all of your perceptions; it beautifies the lens through which you see life.

There have been many men and women through time, who were made to look like fools or lunatics, labeled as such by "the establishment" or world governments, because they attempted to bring better ways of living to light; they had ideas and inventions that would help the masses feel better, be healed, or live more efficiently with less cost. These people were ridiculed, castigated, made to be quacks and shut down, and often left penniless, like Nikola Tesla. As more truth is revealed and unearthed in the 21st Century – which could soon be dubbed the 'century of truth' – people will begin to question those power-hungry entities who may make erroneous claims, and it will hopefully lead to a re-examination of history. Those brilliant minds who were in our midst, who only sought to better and harmonize mankind, but were shut down and humiliated because it would have cost industries and governments billions of dollars in profits, will one day be celebrated and recognized for their contributions to their species; contributions that include such inventions as "free-energy", cancer cures (Royal Rife), and automobiles that do not require a single drop of gasoline, the latter of which came long before the modern electric car, by people whom we were not allowed to fully discover or know about in our modern age.

Even our likeability and attraction to certain colors tells a lot about us and our inner vibrational frequencies; what resonates with us at a given time. Every color has a meaning. During many of my sessions, clients will report seeing a myriad of colors. At times, when my eyes are closed, I see them as well. I sometimes ask the client, if they are not sleeping, whether they had just seen a certain color that flashed before me. Every single time, thus far, they have confirmed that color; it was the same color that they saw or are experiencing. It tells me we are on the same frequency, entraining (merging with a better, healthier energy), blending, and dancing in the same space, assimilating with the same intention and hope. When this occurs, it is a wonderful connection.

Throughout your day, try to slowly focus on your pineal and pituitary glands; those glands that have been, in large part, fast asleep, dormant and recessed in their ebullient capacities. These are powerful glands. The pineal gland, shaped like a core or pineapple, may very well be our antennae to the deepest spiritual part of us – that essence from which we all evolved, and to which we periodically return. Look up the glands. Research them. See what they look like and where they are located in your head. Then, through meditation, focus on them. See them coming back to life and lighting up like light bulbs of the most gorgeous luminance. You may slowly start to experience sensation in your temples, and/or your third eye region. It is part of our 'waking up' process. Enjoy! It is beautiful!

Shed your ego and you start to see yourself, and then you start to see each other, and soon after, whether through an epiphany or arbitrary moment, beauty abounds because you begin to not only understand yourself more, but also the subtleties of that same beauty in everything around you. You see what has been hidden…the *real* you! Ego is a fog that inhibits us. It does not foster progress, but rather, it can nurture alienation and destruction. Ego can be a sign of sub-conscious fear in some people, used as a shield for their insecurities. Bless these people and wish them well. Some of the most powerful people in the world suffer from this, bent on asserting their authority or status, so scared to lose what is theirs, when in reality, nothing is theirs. *Ego* should be listed as a disease, hence, "Oh, he/she is suffering from ego." I have learned that many who are ruled by their own ego lack the precious abil-ity to have empathy, to step outside of themselves and feel for others with sincerity, despite being quite good at saying they do. In the 21st century, their masks will fall off…and we shall all be there to help them, because we are *one*.

I have noticed shifts and differences in the emission of energy and healing, when doing mobile healing (traveling to the client for the session, as opposed to the client coming to me). I already know that my healing room is cleansed, healthy, primed and energized, devoid of negative and impure forces and emotions. However, this is not always the case in other people's homes. In some homes I have immediately sensed a negative draw, whether it be from sorrow, anguish, pain, negativity, trauma, stress, or a litany of other counter-productive emotions. In some cases, I have actually sensed the negative, overbearing, possessing energies of a spouse that in fact only fed and abetted the condition that I was trying to heal! This is something to consider. Be mindful of the space in which you live, and also of the influences therein, from others living with you or coming and going through that space. Focus on harmony and always intend a positive, loving and nurturing space. Also, never forget that positive thoughts are far more powerful than negative thoughts and influences. Smudging with sage or a combination of sage and sweet grass while at the same time intending for love and sanctity in the space, can be helpful. I will repeat a mantra whenever I smudge my space: *I hereby sanctify and cleanse this space. Negative and impure energies do not reside here; they are abolished. Only love and light are here. Love and light! It is thus so! So be it!*

Some people are too immersed in a total and utterly negative workplace and/or lifestyle. I have found that some of these people have difficulty holding onto their healing with any permanence. However, the reasons are rather clear: Their job or situation that is constantly bombarding them with negativity is ever-present in their minds and their bodies. Stress is ever-flowing! It has been my experience that for energy healing to work optimally in its highest degree, *on stress-related ailments and issues*, the subject has to be open to change and to completely receiving the healing; they have to be open to and desiring to be healed, and to ascend to a better place and circumstance. This is free will! Many people know they should get out of their stressful, draining jobs, but cannot, riddled and saddled with re-sponsibility, obligation, and the numbness that comes with the full immersion in the societal program, or sim-ply because they have a family for which to care and provide, all perfectly understandable in this current world. However, do not ever close yourself off to the possibility of change; do not ever feel that there are not any options and that you must drown in your responsibilities like a martyr. You would be doing yourself a great disservice. Many people are too frightened to even acknowledge that there are other options, but there are always options, and they must first be hatched and conceived in the mind. The layers, reasons and complexities behind the resistance to change, can be endless and self-perpetuating. I have had clients for whom I can only provide temporary relief from just *some* of their symptoms, or all of the symptoms but for a very brief duration – one or two days – before they are right back into their stressful environment. These are factors beyond my control and the body will likely respond in the same stressful manner until the habitual situation or mode of employment is changed to something more pleasing to mind, body and soul. For those who might be in similar negative situations, there *is* a way out. It starts in your mind and connects to your heart. Take it one step at a time, be open to new ideas, and let those ideas hatch better visions in your mind. Be patient, yet disciplined. It can be the beginning of striving toward something new, and a lifestyle that is much healthier – the thought of something new alone may bring relief. The duration of each life is but brief, and we are all born with this realization. Therefore, try to avoid the hazards of misery. Try to avoid settling.

Life by nature is not stagnant, but dynamic. Life likes speed and action, and it loses vibrancy with inaction. Perhaps start by choosing to be happy right *now*, regardless of your current circumstance, and resolve to always strive toward and envision happiness. It is a foundation on which to build something better, and your visions of change will likely be equally happy, and attainable.

I once worked as a special education teacher in a very toxic public school environment. There was no support from superiors, and with the rash of recent changes, I believed I could no longer serve children and students as I once had. Teaching, learning, the originality of students, and their individual, inherent talents all hung in the balance as a result of the implementation of the new, vastly cold and impersonal system that espoused a 'one-size-fits-all' educational philosophy. It was deeply bothersome to me. Paperwork increased, and attention to students decreased; I could no longer draw out each student's individual strengths, because the new curriculum demanded all students to be at the same "pre-determined" level of learning and academic cognizance – but those levels were not pre-determined by me, their teacher. This philosophy is in direct contrast to who we are as individual life forces. We are not automatons, but rather vibrant light bodies with original, creative talents and gifts. I began to wonder, "Where will we ever find our next generation of thinkers, geniuses, and creative brilliance? How will we even be able to identify them in this environment?" I humbly admit that one afternoon after school, I came home and sat on my sofa with tears in my eyes, and I said aloud, "I can no longer help and serve my students. It is all out of my hands, in favor of standardized tests and standardized curriculums." My students, having been mainstreamed, were either failing miserably, losing self-esteem, or dropping out of school, and no one seemed to care or notice the trend – even when I tried to speak up. Even worse, I could do nothing about it. I concluded that I was utterly miserable, and I had developed an unhealthy distrust of my superiors who were more concerned with 'toeing the proverbial line' of the system. In my opinion, we had lost our humanity in a human system, and like sheep, everyone obeyed...even the parents of the students. I decided that life was too short and precious to be constantly exposed to toxicity, misery and heartache. I knew that the position was no longer expanding my soul; I was no longer growing as a person, and I felt as though I was in danger of becoming just another worker on 'auto-pilot', who shows up to work, says "yes" to all the new rules and systems, and collects a paycheck. My soul was screaming in rebellion, and I heard it loud and clear. It was all against the grain of who I am – it was against the grain of *me*. I certainly did not become a teacher for the benefits and job security, and thus, regardless of my financial situation, security was secondary in my consideration. I waited until the end of the school year to give my decision serious thought. After the academic year concluded, I deliberated for weeks, weighing pros and cons, assessing the climate for the next school year, and gauging my feelings. Towards the end of the summer, when I received my schedule for the coming school year, I made my decision to resign my position, and promptly submitted my letter of resignation. I then experienced what can happen to a human body that has been under constant stress, and in a toxic environment, when a decision of that magnitude is made. The following week, I became immensely ill – as sick as I've ever been – but it wasn't a virus or ailment, it was a purging and monumental release. My temperature spiked, and I sweated profusely for at least seven consecutive days. I would get up in the middle of the night shivering, and have to change my clothes because they were so drenched I could literally wring them out. I lost my appetite. I lost my strength, and during the days I was pasted to my couch, I slept for long periods, and I sensed as though my body was emptying all of the toxicity, stress and junk that had been accumulated from working at that job for almost five years – it was self-healing. After almost two weeks, I was still weak, although my sweating had decreased. After a few more days, my strength began to come back, and I knew I was on the mend. At that point, I rallied myself and my body back into activity. When I finally made it back to the gym for a workout and stepped on the scale, I was a whole 10 pounds lighter. My skin was fresh and clear. My eyes appeared lighter. It was my own education on the effects that a toxic job can have on a body. I feel that it can be safely deduced that stress and toxicity in the workplace can indeed lead to the steady growth of disease. In my opinion, it's just not worth it. I've always been one to listen to my heart, roll the dice of life, and swim with my soul – that's just who I am, and I realize that not everyone sees life the way I do. Many people are scared that such a decision and life move might cause them to fall. For me, I don't see myself falling…I believe in flying.

Often time, in the midst of healing sessions, I will intend and send sacred geometrical shapes and sacred symbols into the area of focus. I will visualize the symbols, manifest them in my mind's eye, and 'drop' or send them into the spot. I believe it can amplify the healing. I primarily utilize the "Tree of Life", the "Flower of Life", and/or the merkaba, the latter of which is a spiritual vehicle. I visualize all of the shapes in a three-dimensional form, and I add color and detail, all of them always flowing with realness and vitality. For some reason, I almost always see the Tree of Life weaving in the mysteries and whispers of the wind, moving with grace and power. I will also incorporate the U-NAN symbol, featured on page 68, in Alain Herriott's book, *Supercharging Quantum-Touch*, which I highly recommend. In the book, Herriott discusses the colors that comprise healthy cells and cellular patterns.[8]

Merkaba   **Tree of Life**

Flower of Life   **Herriott's U-NAN Symbol**

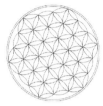   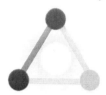

On *Aspartame*, and diet sodas and products containing this ingredient...I was having a business discussion with a woman on the telephone one day, unrelated to energy healing. Somehow, the topic of food and drink snuck into our conversation. I asked her, "You don't drink diet soda do you?" She said that she did. She had at least one full can every day. I told her to stop. The ingredient, *Aspartame*, is not healthy. It is a chemical in the body. She knew nothing about the ingredient. I went on to tell her that there is a correlation between *Aspartame* and many diseases and ailments. A study conducted at the Cesare Maltoni Cancer Research Center of the European Ramazzini Foundation, and published in 2007, concluded that Aspartame increases cancer effects in Rats, and is carcinogenic.[9] A study in the American Journal of Clinical Nutrition claims that men who daily consume multiple soft drinks containing aspartame can bolster their likelihood of having a variety of blood cancers.[10] Our conversation wrapped up, we said our "goodbyes" and I hung up the phone, not expecting to hear from her again. Roughly three weeks later I received a phone call. It was her. "Neal, I am calling to thank you. When we were talking, I did not tell you that for the past six months I have been seeing doctors and dermatologists in an attempt to find the reason and cure for the hives I was getting all over my body. They just started showing up and they were spreading – and they were big! After I spoke to you, I stopped drinking diet soda. Three days later...my hives were gone. I thank *you* for that." In an 'unofficial' study and observation, I have noted that those who consume large amounts of diet soda – four to six cans daily – seem to have a higher incidence of multiple sclerosis, definitive connections and links however, are inconclusive, since I am *not* a scientist. *Aspartame* is not natural. It is not good for the body. It is only another foreign substance added to the bloodstreams. It is in low fat yogurt, soda, some ice cream and frozen treats, and in just about all US-made chewing gum. I went into a Middle Eastern store where I saw them selling *Chicklets* bubble gum. It was made in Lebanon. The ingredients included pure sugar, not *Aspartame.* I order bubble gum that comes from Canada. Again, no *Aspartame.* Only in the United States is *Aspartame* everywhere. Read the ingredients label on the food you buy, and stay away from *Aspartame*. Just because it is in brand name products, products that have become part of the American landscape, does not make it good for you. Drink water, it is the elixir of life – it *is* life.

A healthy body equals healthy energy and optimum energy releases. I had a discussion with a local state representative who wanted to raise taxes on regular soda, (The Soda Tax) so people would consume more diet soda, in an effort to curb obesity and sugar in-take...*and* collect more taxes. I called her on the tele-phone, "Do you realize what you are doing? The regular soda with real sugar is better for you than the *Aspartame* and chemicals in diet soda." She claimed ig-norance and really did not know about the dangers of diet soda. When chemicals like *Aspartame* are ingested, it is hard to know the cause of certain ailments. It be-comes vague and nebulous, like the woman who was experiencing hives. She had seen countless doctors in an effort to find out what caused them. No one could tell her, even after blood tests! In order to set an inten-tion for a healing...it is helpful to know the cause or history of the issue(s). The unconscious ingestion of chemicals can make it very difficult in ascertaining the root of some health issue(s). After all, diet soda drinkers do it out of habit, like smoking. Think about that for a moment. If I hypothetically have a session with a client and succeed in eliminating their symptoms and ailment, but then two hours after they leave me they consume another diet soda, what can be expected based on what we know about habitual lifestyles? Diet soda is a negative energetic substance. A *Webmd.com* 2009 article reported that "Women who drink 2 or more diet sodas daily double their risk of kidney function decline."[11]

Since everything is energy, even the food we consume has a vibrational resonance and frequency. A friend whom I urged to stop using *Splenda*™, another fake sugar substitute which contains sucralose, recently told me that she feels better since she stopped using it. She feels calmer with an improved overall sense of being. *Splenda*™ is allegedly made by *McNeil Pharmaceuticals* – yes, a pharmaceutical company! They have recently attempted to repackage the product to compete with the more natural *Stevia*. Beware of engineered foods. If it is not of the earth – or the natural universe for that matter – then it is not natural to you. As we continue to evolve, we will become more aware of the vibrational resonance of the food that we consume; we will be aware of the energy signature or 'wholesomeness' of the food we eat. We must give more attention to what we feed our bodies, and start to demand better choices. Perhaps one day in our evolved future, diets might consist of pure light, for we would be feeding that which we are – we are light beings…it is just that many have forgotten and/or fail to realize it. I am uncertain how far off this 'diet of light' might be, but in my active imagination I have my hopes, and as a healer, I can frankly see its possibilities. Ironically, as I write this, food portions are getting smaller and the price of meat has reached record highs in the United States.

Collective mind can affect the earth and its entire people. If the majority of humanity can somehow find a way to stay in a positive energetic mindset, one that does not give power to fear, doubt and worry, but instead stays in the present moment and focuses with gratitude and elation to those empowering, innate, positive attributes within, we can together change the world, wrestling control away from the few, and giving it to all! We *do* have the power to reset the global societal program. Unity in energy can heal not only an earth, but an entire population of people and shift the frequency of everyone, all at once. Author Lynne McTaggart has written about this in her books that discuss in great detail verifiable experiments that were conducted. What frequency are you on? Is it positive or negative? Intend a good one. *Choose to be happy and manifest a great reality now!*

GMO (genetically modified organisms), are on the rise, as companies and corporate conglomerates seek to infiltrate our foods and our diets with unnatural substances to feed – and perhaps control – the burgeoning population. It is clear that there are many who do wish to take control of how we conduct our lives, and they are going right to the source – our genes – altering the food we consume and thereby, within a generation, altering us as human beings. Yes, there are those that are *trying* to play God. How is this to be handled? I find myself repeating a particular statement aloud, more and more: *Not in my world; not in my reality.* Remember, what we think about we bring about. If we are fearful of these companies who are trying to engineer our foods and violating the laws of nature, we only serve to empower them and embolden their efforts, because 'fear' is a weakened position and a form of control; 'fear' is a *dis*empowering form of energy and one of low vibration. We must not focus on our fears, but rather on our strengths and solutions. Thus, while I stay *aware* of the headlines pertaining to this subject, I do not *digest* them. I counter them with healthy thoughts of the world that I desire, that in turn makes me feel good, which only accelerates the process of bringing it to me, in full, emblazoned manifestation! I also might become more knowledgeable about sustainable living practices as a solution, in order to spread *that* self-sufficient, independent energy, and align myself with people of similar sentiment. We are in the midst of experiencing a split in our reality on this earth; a duality of high frequency and high vibration, with low frequency and low vibration. Which one feels better? Which one will be yours? Choose – and think – wisely. These times in which we currently live are ripe. They are some of the most unique times to ever occur in the concourse of human history, clearly demonstrated and played out in world headlines. Stay away from engineered foods…but do not dwell on them. Visualize and feel the perfect world for you. Then be patient, take small actions to make it come about, starting with feelings of joy and happiness, regardless of your present circumstance. Be confident in your expectations…and watch them unfold.

When you watch television, turn OFF the drug and pharmaceutical commercials. They are intended to leave subliminal impressions on your subconscious; impressions of disease and adverse health conditions. People who do not know any better may begin asking internal questions and making statements detrimental to their well-being: *Do I have that condition? Should I ask my doctor about that drug? If I have that condition, is this a drug for me? If I get that disease now I know what to take.* Big pharma makes billions off of your thoughts; off of thoughts of fear and the dreaded 'fight or flight' response. It is in the adverse, negative energy of the message that penetrates and circulates through the living areas of your home, and into the depths of your conscience and subconscious, where, if the message is strong enough, it could manifest from there. Remember, our bodies obey our thoughts very well...and so does our reality, which is the raw blueprint of our manifested thoughts. The evidence is all around you.

Very soon, for those who continue to prescribe and act according to 20th century thoughts, belief patterns and behaviors, the universe will no longer respond to them. They will thus be forced to accept the new and healthier ways of the 21st century. A new, buoyant and more fulfilling female energy is bombarding the planet right now, and it will soon affect every single soul. You may already be noticing subtle changes around you, and in our national and global landscape. I am confident that the 21st century will *eventually* be defined by harmony, and even pure love. While it may be a bumpy ride until we get there, embrace it all. A new hope is here.

It is important to also bear in mind that even social and civil upheaval can be part of the natural progression toward *eventually* healing a civilization. I add this here in lieu of the social and ideological strife and violence that has been grabbing headlines around the world. Try not to examine these episodes in part, but rather as a whole; avoid a microcosmic viewpoint, and instead employ a *macro*cosmic view. Ask questions: *How did we get here? How might this be part of our collective evolution? Are these headlines mere propaganda that are part of a larger agenda?* Try not to let the episode(s) hinder, inhibit or dampen your reality and energy – however difficult it may sometimes be. Be grateful for the contrast of extremes that it offers. A reality shift can merely – and simply – be a shift in perception. We are living in very rare, but volatile times, but every bit of it is energy, with an energetic cause and effect. For those who may be prescribing to, and/or committing sinister acts or orchestrating sinister agendas around the globe, they are damaging their own karma, as well as detracting from their own human species – which goes beyond *any* religion. It shall be 'recorded' on their soulful balance sheet, as something to repay and serve as a 'life lesson'.

For those who think this life is long, I believe each of the next three will be even longer, and thus…consider those potential consequences, of living three successive longer lives riddled with negative karmic repercussions; it could be a relative purgatory. This is the 'boomerang effect'. What we put out…*always* comes back.

On sacred contracts…sometimes, despite the best medical care and healing powers, people still transition and pass on, and loved ones ask, *why?* Sometimes, it is simply because they decided to do so, in that chosen or destined hour, long before they got here and incarnated. It is a higher sacred contract, and in this life, we all have a role and/or lesson to complete. So…if you're still reading this, your purpose – and contract – is not yet done or fulfilled, because if it was you would likely already have passed over. However, I do absolutely believe that we all reunite in the 'in-between', as in, *Hey…I'll meet you back here soon*. For the most part, I believe this life is part classroom and part video game, but we *do* get to design many details of the game, much like the movie *The Matrix*.

If more people would consciously desire and intend to open their minds, awaken its long dormant chambers and expand their ability to imagine, life itself would take on much more color and meaning, replete with new ideas and an insight previously absent. Through the activation of the imagination, the ways in which we as a people have lived as conformists to society, and spent our time for the past hundred years and beyond, would slowly and increasingly become apparent, and in some ways…it would be viewed as trite, restricted and shallow, but there should be gratitude for such revelations because they provide us with a measure of the extremes; sweet with the sour, tasty with the bland, enlightenment against darkness, which results in growth. We now have the capacities on a mass level to see the difference between where we are, and where we can go. It starts in the mind. Everyone has the ability to imagine. Try it and watch what you slowly begin to create. It is where every idea that has ever been hatched, was first born.

Contrary to what many news headlines may portray, there is *always* hope! I urge you all to get on this frequency…the *frequency of hope*. And remember, happiness is a choice. Be alert. Be informed. Seek solutions to issues and act on them in accordance to your convictions, but stay hopeful amidst it all. We are indeed living in volatile times, but I believe that the more resistance there 'appears' to be, only means that we as a global people are that much closer to something better. I also believe that if all of the people – the citizens of this great world – got together and intended to positively heal humanity and the planet, on the same frequency, with the same loving intentions, nothing could control us; nothing could have dominion over us. The energy of us as *One* would be too great to overcome, and it would likely be seen from deep space – seriously! *That's* how powerful we really are.

In this plane of existence, that which we cannot see is far more powerful than that which we can see. It always will be. The real power is in unseen space, not in the objects around you that are in the 'perceived' physical space. All that you perceive as material is just an illusion – *things* that you have willed and manifested into your life; a reality that *you* have created. It is all evidence of the power you have, that we all have within us. The proof of the power of your thoughts is all around you! Smile, it is all quite beautiful, just as you are.

You are *not* your body. You are *spirit*! You are *light*! You are *love*! You are *not* your worries. You are *not* your guilt. You are definitely *not* your fears. You are *now*!

You are here, reading these words, in this moment, pulsating with life. Embrace your breaths and imagine a higher place…this is the place from where you come. Be *you* and go within. Dally and dance! The answers and your true freedom are all there. You are loved!

Be mindful of what kind of space you create – the very space in which you live and work. Become sensitive to it. Within any space is energy. Take safeguards to ensure that you are in a positively charged, high vibrational space. It ought to be ever-welcoming to you… and also to those around you. I have received numerous compliments on the space where I conduct my healing sessions. Visitors and clients feel a sense of calm, tranquility and peace, which makes perfect sense – it is the space that is constantly charged with love, healing, and care. Conversely, you should avoid those spaces that you sense are toxic, or are of a low vibrational frequency, i.e. places where negative, desperate or nefarious activities occur; or anger, hatred and abuse, for they can be vastly unhealthy for countless reasons, and like ethereal barbs, sometimes this low energy can stick to unsuspecting personal, bodily energy fields, resulting in a fatiguing drain. As an example, just think of how you felt after being in a place you didn't want to be, or sensed you didn't belong because of low or negative energy, it could even be a toxic workplace environment. Perhaps you may have even experienced this around particular individuals, of whom you just didn't feel right being near them. You may have been sensing their negative energy, and the reasons for your sensations may even extend beyond this life…to those long past. The memories of your soul are endless – it is your compass.

If we all live in harmony, the world will be in harmony. Please seek this harmony. If you seek in earnest, it will be yours and the path getting there…will seem magical!

There are indeed certain wounds that simply cannot be healed; that require a frequency not yet present on this earth, but one, I have surmised, that could be on its way through the continual evolution of our planet and of our species, in our ever-evolving solar system and galaxy. Frequency…is a word that I urge the masses to comprehend and grasp, for it can and will one day cure and heal everything that requires or needs healing.

I believe we can birth our next lives with our thoughts, visualizations, and actions in this life. Remember, we live in a quantum reality. This notion is espoused and explored in the movie, *Cloud Atlas*, a lengthy film, but one that I highly recommend for further understanding of this concept.

Surrender to the gravity of life. It will flow much better. Try to resist the desire to control and manipulate situations.

Envision a better world – and *hold* that vision steadfast in your mind!

In conjunction with energy healing, I will often suggest holistic remedies or natural applications. The three I most often recommend are topical castor oil packs, apple cider vinegar, and ginger root. Besides being excellent complements to most diet regimens, they contain numerous healing properties. I recommend reading up on Edgar Cayce, who widely prescribed castor oil packs for a variety of ailments (beware that castor oil can stain clothes and fabric). Apple cider vinegar is remarkable for staving off colds and flu and maintaining vitality, and I have had personal success using it to help dissolve kidney stones. I typically recommend mixing 1 to 2oz of apple cider vinegar, to 10 to 12oz of water. I will then use flavored liquid stevia drops to sweeten into a cool drink, or I will heat the ingredients on a stove with cinnamon, pour into a mug, add liberal amounts of honey, stir and enjoy. Other natural remedies I will suggest to clients based on varying conditions: turmeric, garlic, cayenne pepper, coconut oil and honey, the latter of which can be extremely effective all by itself. The earth beneath our feet can be a worthy, positively-charged medicine cabinet. Please research these remedies on your own before trying them, and consult with a homeopathic physician and/or competent medical professional for specified guidance. This information is based on my own personal experiences.

Energy healing is excellent for pets. I have had success applying energy healing to cats, who are sensitive to healing frequencies. I have also seen it successfully applied to other animals. There is an excellent video on *YouTube* from the *Earthfire Institute: Wildlife Sanctuary and Retreat Center* that demonstrates the healing of a wolf in the wild. The video is entitled, "Energy Healing Wolf", and I highly recommend viewing it.

The two greatest expressions in the English language: *Thank you* and *I love you*! Say them as often as possible. The positive energy emitted through both, is immeasurable...and it all comes back to you tenfold. Love is the butterfly of your heart, for when it flutters, our wings open up and we soar. Yearn to discover new moments of your soul in flight.

One day, we will all be gathered in a place *other* than earth, and we will talk about and marvel over how we lived life now, in these times. Great change is underway, and though it may get darker before it gets lighter, it is only so no one will ever again forget the difference between the extremes. Love to you all.

We are all energy. Energy cannot be created or destroyed and thus, we cannot be destroyed. As an article published in *Scientific American* explained:

> The law of conservation of energy, also known as the first law of thermodynamics, states that the energy of a closed system must remain constant—it can neither increase nor decrease without interference from outside. The universe itself is a closed system, so the total amount of energy in existence has always been the same. The forms that energy takes, however, are constantly changing.[12]

There is no end. We keep going. Perhaps we shall meet in the next life. Until then…Godspeed. We are all magnificent. In love and light always – I thank you.

If you have questions that pertain to any of the content in this book, or if you wish to schedule an energy healing session, I can be reached through my website: **www.QuantumEnergyTreatment.com**

*** Mention this book and receive your first session at half the regular rate.*

** Please also visit and *"Like"* my *Facebook* page **"The Age of Healing: Profiles from an Energy Healer"**, where I will be posting periodic videos, messages and other information, including occasional contests to get a **FREE session** by me.

As mentioned in the beginning of this book, I am certified in *Quantum-Touch*™ energy healing. There are many modalities of healing, and inevitably, it is what works for you – it is what resonates most, feels most comfortable, etc. There may be many rooms in a large house, but they are all under the same roof. If you wish to become a practitioner, explore the modality in which I am certified, or even learn more about energy healing, you may visit: **www.QuantumTouch.com**

Bibliographical Notes

1. Henry, R. C. (2005). The mental universe. *Nature*, 436, 29-29. doi:10.1038/436029a

2. Corinthians 4:16-18 New International Version. (n.d.). Retrieved March 13, 2015, from bible.com/bible/111/2co.4.16-18.niv

3. Virtue, D. (2007). Three - Mind and matter. In *The Lightworkers Way: Awakening your Spiritual Power to Know and Heal* (p. 21). London: Hay House.

4. Gallup, G., & Proctor, W. (1982). *Adventures in Immortality*. New York: McGraw-Hill.

5. Lanza, R., M.D. (2011, November 19). Is death an illusion? Evidence suggests death isn't the end. Retrieved from robertlanzabiocentrism.com/is-death-an-illusion-evidence-suggests-death-isnt-the-end/

6. Petrov, A. (2011). *Creation of the Universe: Save Yourself.* Hamburg: Jelezky.

7. Stress management. (2014, March 4). *Mayo Clinic.* Retrieved from mayoclinic.org/healthy-living/stress-management/in-depth/positive-thinking/art-20043950?pg=2

8. Herriott, A. (2007). *Supercharging Quantum-Touch: Advanced Techniques.* Berkeley, CA: North Atlantic Books.

9. Soffritti, M., Belpoggi, F., Tibaldi, E., Esposti, D. D., &Lauriola, M. (2007, June 13). Life-Span exposure to low doses of aspartame beginning during prenatal life increases cancer effects in rats. Retrieved from ncbi.nlm.nih.gov/pmc/articles/PMC1964906/

10. Chavarria, L. (2013, October 25). Diet soda dangers: New study may link aspartame to cancer. *Fox 32 News*. Retrieved from myfoxchicago.com/ story/20939173/diet-soda-dangers-new-study-may-link-aspartame-to-cancer

11. Doheny, K., & Chang, L., M.D. (2009, November 2). Diet sodas may be hard on the kidneys. *WebMD*. Retrieved from webmd.com/diet/ 20091102/diet-sodas-hard-on-the-kidneys

12. Moskowitz, C. (2014, August 5). Fact or fiction?: Energy can neither be created nor destroyed. *Scientific American*. Retrieved from scientificamerican.com/article/ energy-can-neither-be-created-nor-destroyed/

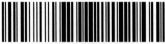